Celestial Secrets

A Dūnhuáng Manuscript of Medicinal Decoctions for the *Zàngfǔ* Organs

Praise for Celestial Secrets

"The introduction is a remarkably interesting dive into the history of both the *Tangye Jing* and the *Fuxing Jue*, which Wilms demonstrates is a medieval text of historical significance rather than a modern forgery. But the reader is also treated to a meeting with the colorful Daoist Tao Hongjing, Master of Maoshan and compiler of the *Collected Commentaries on the Divine Farmer's Classic of Materia Medica*. And all this is *before* arriving at the lucid and practical translation of the *Fuxing Jue* (including Chinese characters) together with useful commentary and explanation (including diagrams and illustrations) by Sharon Weizenbaum. Overall, a book I can't wait to have on my bookshelf!"

—Steve Clavey, author of *Fluid Physiology and Pathology in Traditional Chinese Medicine* and editor at *The Lantern*

"A brilliant piece of detective work! I really enjoyed reading it! I find it well-balanced in perspectives, meticulously argued and rigorously substantiated. An immensely helpful guide for clinicians who have hitherto not been exposed to the methods of textual bibliography and analysis. This is an ingenious use of a high-interest text to showcase the tools of philology for locating the text in the historical timeline."

—Leo Lok, LAc, founder of *Voices of Our Medical Ancestors*

"This small, readable, remarkably unpretentious book is several texts in one: For dedicated clinicians, it is the first published English translation of the *Fuxingjue* — including the text sometimes referred to as the *Tangyejing* — which invites us to look at herb dynamics in relation to the 5 phases. For scholar-practitioners, Sabine's philological work is impeccable, helping us to understand the detective work of translating early Chinese texts, and how exactly they can be dated through word usage and other clues. Additionally, the book is just a great read — entertaining, even suspenseful, not unlike Jonathan Spence's living histories — it's a story that is fun to curl up with and hard to put down."

—Claudia Citkovitz, PhD, MS, LAc,
director of Acupuncture Services, NYU Langone Hospital, Brooklyn, and author of *Acupressure and Acupuncture During Birth*

"Sabine Wilms has once again provided English readers with a beautiful and important translation of a text shrouded in mystery and a source for great interest in both the East and the West. Its importance in understanding the development of classical formulas and classical methods, especially in the proper historical context, which Dr. Wilms has so thoroughly provided in the introduction, cannot be understated. For this, anyone with interest in these subjects should sit with a good cup of tea and slowly and mindfully devour its pages. Sabine's translation style is both poetic and historically accurate, and once again, she has delivered with this rendition of the *Fu Xing Jue*."

—Eran Even, PhD, DrTCM, translator of *Formulas from the Golden Cabinet with Songs, Volumes IV-VI*.

"Wilms offers not only a reliable translation of the *Fǔxíngjué*, but also introduces the history of the text in a way that practitioners, scholars, and students alike will find accessible and interesting. She is one of a very small number of historically-trained translators of Chinese medical texts who have the knowledge to do justice to this text."

—Pierce Salguero, PhD, Associate Professor of Asian History & Religious Studies and Program Chair for Interdisciplinary Studies, The Abington College of Penn State University; Editor in Chief of *Asian Medicine: Journal of the International Association for the Study of Traditional Asian Medicine*; and author of the *Buddhism & Medicine* series from Columbia University Press

"As a long-time admirer of Sabine Wilms' work and two decades long devoted student of Sharon Weizenbaum's teachings on Classical Chinese Medicine, I am thrilled to see this project combining their talents as translator-historian and scholar-physician. This previously unavailable-in-English translation and commentary on the *Fuxingjue* has both historical and clinical significance and I was captivated by Dr Wilms' Chinese History Train that both demystified and contextualized this poorly understood text. Incredibly well sourced, this text expands confining concepts into broader implications of cosmic circular dynamics and lends another lens to familiar formulas. They are giving a great gift to students of Chinese history and clinicians alike."

—Caroline Radice, DACM, LAc, NCCAOM, Vice President of the Shen Nong Society)

"For years I've been fascinated by the idea that a precursor text to the *Shanghanlun* called the *Tangyejing* existed. I've seen supposed excerpts from it here and there, but I could never figure out why some claimed to have it and others said that there were no existing copies. I am so excited and grateful to Sabine Wilms and Sharon Weizenbaum for bringing forth this translation and unraveling the mystery behind the *Tangyejing* and the related text the *Fuxingjue*. The fascinating story behind the connection between these texts is told with great thoroughness and imagination by Sabine.

The translation itself with commentary by Sharon will be so useful to every clinician interested in *Shanghanlun* formulas and their modifications. One of the values of this text is that it illustrates the connection between the *wu xing* (5 phases) underlying qualities of an integral group of individual herbs. This group of herbs are the most fundamental used in classical formulas, and the historical significance of this shift in perspective is explained via the lineage of medical literature. As a clinician myself, I particularly value how Sharon explains the dynamics of each formula in terms of the directions and the constellations. This will not only deepen your understanding of formulas and disease dynamics for your patients, but it will also enhance your experience of our human interaction with the cosmos."

—Sally Rappeport, LAc, Founder & President,
Shen Nong Society)

"Dr. Sabine Wilms is a great gift to Chinese Medicine. Her translations are known for their clarity and readability, while providing the proper historical and contextual perspective of the source material. In this latest book, she takes the reader on a fascinating journey that explores the origins of the *Fǔxíngjué* manuscript and brings to life the ancient formulas that work with the movement of the stars. This book is excellent and I learned some important things, which always makes me happy!"

—Lillian Bridges,
author of *Face Reading in Chinese Medicine*)

"The legendary history of its discovery and the controversy over the authenticity of the editions have given this medical manuscript an additional mystical flavor. In my perspective, though, it is ultimately not important whether the *Fǔxíngjué zàngfǔ yòngyào fǎyào* is authentic or a forgery. What is important is whether it has value in clinical application. The description of the fifty plus formulas and patterns in this text and the plain writing style, which are certainly not randomly composed, suggest that it is the work of a clinician. As such, it is entirely possible to view this text as a commentary on Zhāng Zhòngjǐng's classical formulas."

—Prof. Huáng Huáng 黄煌, dean of the International Jing Fang Institute of Nanjing University of Chinese Medicine, author of *Ten Key Formula Families in Chinese Medicine* and countless other books.

"As western practitioners of Chinese medicine, we often run up against the barriers of not just modern Chinese language but also classical Chinese characters and philosophy. As such, we are indebted to the translators who offer us a glimpse at the texts that form the backbone of this medicine. Once again, Sabine has given our profession both an insightful translation and a thought-provoking discussion. To what depths are we willing to take our scholarship, and how do we pass on this knowledge? We are in the midst of a translation renaissance of Chinese medicine and Daoist thought, and I am confident that Sabine and her translations will continue to be a guiding force in our understanding of Classical Chinese medicine."

—Robert Hoffman, DAOM, LAc, Dean, DAOM Program, Yo San University of Traditional Chinese Medicine

"The *Fuxing Jue* has long been shrouded in mystery, and I've heard and read various accounts of its origins, loss, rediscovery, association with the lost *Tangye Jing*, etc. Here we have the most comprehensive accounting of the when, what, who and why's of this text that I've ever encountered. Sabine Wilms' translation of the *Fuxing Jue* is - as is true of all her work - far more than simply a translation. Dr. Wilms situates the reader in the context which magnifies the relevance of the text. I believe her goal in demystifying the text is not to diminish its importance, but rather to calibrate its impact with a rigorous understanding of where it stands in its relationship to other works.

Dr. Wilms' deliberate and meticulous choice of terminology, and justifications of her choices, triggers epiphanies we didn't know we needed, and has real implications in how we understand passages and formulas. For example, translating *dan* as a verb rather than a noun ("dawning" rather than "dawn" in the Minor and Major Formulas of the Two Yáng and Yīn Dàn Decoctions) helps us situate the functions of these formulas with the birth periods of Yin and Yang rather than with the literal dawn of the day. As a clinician whose primary focus over the last decade has been the study and application of the *Shanghan Zabing Lun*, I appreciate this work immensely because it too provides a certain context for Zhang Zhongjing's writings. This context can be understood not only by knowing which other works informed its writing, but also by knowing which other works existed within the same sphere, descendants of a common ancestor, and shedding light on the thinking of an era that has long passed."

—Phil Settels, LAc, MSTCM, Dean of Academic Affairs, Academy of Chinese Culture and Health Sciences

"Sabine's love of medicine, history, and old Chinese shines through in all her works, but this one is different because it is a detective story as well. The 湯液經 *Tangyejing* is a "lost" text that has haunted herbalists for thousands of years. As mythic as it is in its influence, it's also problematic, as Chinese doctors like to be able to trace and track their influences and references for their thinking and commentaries. And the *Tangyejing* is curiously missing in terms of tangible goods. Its history is troubled to say the least.

Dr. Wilms is noted for her lively way of blending scholarship with poetry, historical context with modern perspectives, and for her keen eye towards detail and distilling out not just the clinically valuable information from ancient texts, but at the same time enlivening the material in a way that makes it readily accessible to the present-day practitioner.

This translation of the *Fuxingjue,* along with the history of this document as told through the eyes and mind of a studied historian of our medicine, will not only give you a new glimpse into Zhang Zhongjing's formulations. Through the commentary of Sharon Weizenbaum, it also provides a helpful clinical perspective on human physiology as seen through the lens of the 六經 *liùjīng* ("Six Conformations"). This view not only is helpful in better understanding herbal medicine, it furthermore will allow you to better grasp the cycles of qi transformation that will aid in diagnostic and treatment choices as well. There have been bits and snippets concerning the *Tangyejing* scattered through the historical writings of our medicine, but here in *Celestial Secrets: A Dunhuang Manuscript of Medicinal Decoctions for the Zangfu Organs* you'll find perhaps the most comprehensive rendering of the history of this mythic text, along with valuable perspectives on herbal medicine that you can bring into your modern clinical work."

—Michael Max, LAc, host of the *Qiological* podcast

ALSO BY SABINE WILMS

Channeling the Moon
A Translation and Discussion of Qí Zhòngfǔ's
Hundred Questions on Gynecology
齊仲甫《女科百問》
Part One • Questions 1 – 14
Part Two • Questions 15 – 50

Humming with Elephants
A Translation and Discussion of *Sù Wèn 5*
(Great Treatise on the Resonant Manifestations of Yin and Yang)
《黃帝內經，素問：陰陽應象大論篇第五》

The Divine Farmer's Classic of Materia Medica
《神農本草經》 *Shén Nóng Běncǎo Jīng*

Twelve Characters:
A Transmission of Wang Fengyi's Teachings
《王鳳儀十二字薪傳》

Let the Radiant Yang Shine Forth:
Lectures on Virtue by Liu Yousheng
劉有生《演講錄》

Venerating the Root:
Sun Simiao's *Bei Ji Qian Jin Yao Fang*,
Volume 5 on Pediatrics • Parts One and Two
孫思邈《備急千金要方》

Celestial Secrets

A Dūnhuáng Manuscript of Medicinal Decoctions for the *Zàngfǔ* Organs

Translation of the

《輔行訣臟腑用藥法要》

Fǔxíngjué Zàngfǔ Yòngyào Fǎyào

(Secret Tips for Helpful Action: The Key to Using Medicinals on the *Zàngfǔ* Organs)

Sabine Wilms, PhD

HAPPY GOAT PRODUCTIONS
WHIDBEY ISLAND WA • USA

Published by Happy Goat Productions
Whidbey Island, WA • USA

To purchase our books, visit:
HappyGoatProductions.com/onlinestore

Published in the United States of America

First published in 2020

ISBN 978-1-7321571-7-0

Foreword and additional commentary with illustrations by Sharon Weizenbaum, LAc,
Director of White Pine Healing Arts — whitepinehealingarts.org

Cover Photo by Hidenori Tada
www.instagram.com @go_frame1

Additional cover art – front: detail from a star map from around 700 CE, discovered at Dūnhuáng; back: The four Spirit Guardians of the Directions & detail from manuscript cover of the *Fǔxíngjué* from 1964.

Book Design by Barbara Tada
www.pixelgardendesign.com

Dedication

To the ancients
who knew

how to…
howl with the wolves
wiggle with the earthworm
swim with the salmon
dance with the fireflies
sing with the orcas
taste the full moon's dew
tread the Big Dipper
and listen to the cedar.

To those who remember

And to those who are learning

And to my old dog Mr. Nilson, sweetest of the sweet.

Contents

Foreword

By Sharon Weizenbaum

I AM HONORED TO INTRODUCE THIS excellent translation and commentary on the *Fǔxíngjué*, and to provide a clinician's perspective. I have a long relationship with Dr. Sabine Wilms' visionary translation work, and also with this text, which has for many years both fascinated me and haunted me. Its origins are shrouded in mystery, and its content is rich, though contradictory and confusing at times. Dr. Wilms' careful historical and philological work dispels much of the fog regarding its contents and its placement in history.

When the origins of a text are unknown, it is like mist that obscures the base of a mountain, showing viewers only its peaks but making the shape and terrain of the base invisible. In this situation, the book is vulnerable to extravagant and exotic misperceptions on the basis of what appears to the modern eye, unless readers and translators are careful to probe the misty trails with straightforward questions. This investigation is what Dr. Wilms undertakes here, with the meticulous attention to detail belonging to a true scholar of classical Chinese language, history, and culture.

The sacred texts known as the "canons" or "classics" of traditional East Asian medicine, such as the *Huángdì nèijīng* 黃帝內經 (Yellow Emperor's Inner Classic), *Nànjīng* 難經 (Classic of Difficulties), *Shénnóng běncǎojīng* 神農本草經 (Divine Farmer's Classic of Materia Medica), and *Yìjīng* 易經 (Classic of Changes), hold a special status for practitioners of East Asian Medicine. They are regarded as foundational edicts: decrees and precepts that our profession has collectively, for roughly two thousand years, agreed to build upon rather than question. The Chinese term for "classic" is 經 *jīng*, which also means "warp," a technical term in weaving that describes the long, strong anchoring threads around which the wefts, or 緯 *wěi*, are woven. In literature, including medical literature, classics represent the *jīng*, and the texts arising from and held together by the *jīng* are the *wěi*, the weft. Because the classics are *jīng*, we clinicians read them in a particular and humble manner: They are contemplated, chewed on, pondered, turned over and over in our minds and hearts. Our practice is to assume that, if something doesn't make sense, the fault is ours: We have not yet penetrated its meaning, and so we ruminate onward. I have often had the experience with the *Huángdì nèijīng*, as well as the *Dàodéjīng* 道德經 (Classic of the Way and its Potency) and the *Yìjīng* (Classic of Change), of it not making sense and not making sense and then — suddenly it makes perfect sense.

It is a fundamental quality of our medicine that canonical texts are meditated on and worked with over time like this. Who decides if a text is a classic? Though the inclination is understandable, it cannot be based on the unilateral hunch or wish of a non-historian. The texts we regard as canons or classics are specifically those that have earned the nomenclature through this humbly devoted study, agreed upon by the countless generations of clinicians and scholars since the Hàn dynasty.

Wěi books have always been open to questioning, in ways that the *Huángdì nèijīng* and other canonical texts are not. To authenticate and date a found text, we depend on historians and philologists like Dr. Wilms. Later texts are always interpretations of classical principles; they cannot be anything else. This includes influential texts written by such greats as Lǐ Dōngyuán 李東垣, Zhāng Jǐngyuè 張景岳, and Sūn Sīmiǎo 孫思邈, who, while deeply respected, have been argued about and questioned extensively and productively over time. When we turn their writing over and over if it's confusing, contrived, not useful, or even bogus, we can toss out parts that don't fit or don't make sense to us — or elaborate on ones that are clinically useful.

The contents of the *Fǔxíngjué* do have roots in canonical texts, just as all of our traditional medical texts do. It is the nature of all *wěi* ("weft") texts to be connected to the *jīng* (warp) texts. A danger of regarding a *wěi* text as *jīng* is that it may hinder clinicians' own critical thinking, stifling open scrutiny of its accuracy or clinical value. Unilateral canonization of a later piece of writing such as the *Fǔxíngjué* should be regarded with a critical eye and with a query as to what might be the long-term or immediate results of student-practitioners taking the humbly uncritical stance traditionally reserved for *jīng*.

The *Fǔxíngjué* is claimed, by the grandson of the man who supposedly purchased it, to have been found in the Dūnhuáng caves in 1904. However, unlike other Dūnhuáng manuscripts, this discovery cannot be substantiated by that original text's existence. After reportedly being found, it was then reportedly lost again, though memorized by a single person and then dictated from memory more than fifty years later. The dictation was recorded in no less than twenty-one slightly differing manuscripts, all now known as the *Fǔxíngjué*. Chinese linguists, archaeologists, and historians have studied these manuscripts. Their consensus is that, even taking the gap in provenance into consideration, the contents could not have been originally written before the sixth century CE. In the present book, Dr. Wilms agrees with these experts and provides compelling arguments why the text is likely to have come from among the Dūnhuáng manuscripts and date to between the sixth and tenth centuries CE.

When I first studied the material of the *Fǔxíngjué* many years ago, it was presented to me as a part of the lost classic, the *Tāngyèjīng* 湯液經 ("Classic of Decoctions"). I was taught that this supposedly classical material was the theoretical foundation and historical predecessor of Zhāng Zhòngjǐng's 張仲景 *Shānghán zábìng lùn* 傷寒雜病論 (Treatise on Cold Damage and Miscellaneous Diseases). As such, it was promoted as essential foundational knowledge to obtain if one was to understand classical formulas properly. As its name shows, this so-called *Tāngyèjīng*, if it existed, was a "classic." As a non-existent text, it is a perfect blank screen onto which to project a book such as the *Fǔxíngjué*, if one should so desire. And, dressing a *wěi* text up as a *jīng* text imbues the material with a kind of unquestionable power that a simply very thought-provoking medieval book would not have. However, in its essence, the instruction I was receiving about the material in the *Fǔxíngjué* did not make sense to me as a clinician. In large part, this was because its contents, especially the sections on the *zàng* organ formulas, which comprise the bulk of the book, and the twenty-five herbal ingredients organized according to the five phases, though compelling, did not fit well with my knowledge of the classics nor of the *Shānghán zábìng lùn*. Though the *Huángdì nèijīng* associates flavors with the *wǔxíng* 五行 ("five phases"), the attribution of actual herbs and then formulas to the *wǔxíng* was absent from medical literature until the Sòng dynasty. Indeed, Zhāng Zhòngjǐng himself never referred to the *wǔxíng* as any kind of guiding principle for his formulas, nor did he cite the *Tāngyèjīng* when naming the books that had influenced him.

My own experience as clinician is that the ideas of the *Fǔxíngjué*, though enlightening and powerful, are not essential to the mastery of classical formulas. Indeed, I have studied with notable contemporary *jīngfāng* masters such as Huáng Huáng 黄煌, Fù Yánlíng 傅延龄 and Féng Shìlún 冯世纶, who did not consider this material helpful to understanding *jīngfāng*. The idea that the material in the

Fŭxíngjué was the foundation of Zhāng Zhòngjǐng's theory just did not correlate. In addition, this absence of mention of the *Tāngyèjīng* in important medical texts is consistent throughout history. The *Tāngyèjīng*, unlike all other classical texts, which are regularly cited by later authors such as Zhāng Zhòngjǐng, Lǐ Dōngyuán, and many others repeatedly throughout history, is noticeably absent.

Dr. Wilms' work here, by illuminating the facts, has lent harmony and coherence to my understanding by placing the *Fŭxíngjué* in its historical context. Not only does it make more sense, this has also rescued me from passing on misinformation. For me, the publication of her translation and commentary offers a clear example of how important it is for us clinicians to communicate with historians in order to examine, with their help, the genuine historical sources of what we are taught. With the *Fŭxíngjué* given its proper historical place, we can now join Dr. Wilms on her exploration of this powerful material.

The *Fŭxíngjué* is a compilation of six sections, most of which focus on formulas to supplement and drain the *zàng* organs. These sections and the one on the twenty-five herbs are the ones that particularly date the text as having been created no earlier than the sixth century. Nevertheless, the section on the six spirit and dawning formulas is of a very different nature. These formulas are strikingly similar, and in some cases identical to, formulas of the *Shānghánlùn*. Additionally, the names of some of the formulas, such as the Major and Minor Green-Blue Dragon Decoctions and the White Tiger Decoctions are the same as formula names in the *Shānghánlùn*. Though we can be certain that the *Fŭxíngjué* as a whole was compiled no earlier than the sixth century, this particular section resonates with and probably has origins in much more ancient times. These formulas have always fascinated me, and so I have added my own commentary on their clinical value to Wilms's historical commentary in the Translation section of this book.

In the following pages, Dr. Wilms takes us on a wonderful journey through the history and language of our predecessors. We learn here not only about the *Fǔxíngjué* but also about the fascinating academic process linguists and historians go through to determine the origins of written text. I want to take this opportunity to give appreciation to Dr. Wilms and to the academic scholars of Chinese language and history, such as Paul Unschuld, Ma Jixing, Vivienne Lo, Elisabeth Hsu, and many more who are not sufficiently read by most practitioners of Chinese medicine. Scholars like these are our partners and, in some ways, our protectors. We clinicians need them, or we can be led astray.

It may seem strange to be encouraging the reader to not attribute too much importance to a text I am writing the foreword to! However, we can only obtain the real value of this book if we know its place. Though it is important to distinguish the *jīng* "warp" from the *wěi* "weft," a text does not have to be a *jīng* to have great value. Dr. Wilms, having shown us where to place the *Fǔxíngjué* historically, invites us to now engage the text as to its value for us as clinicians. This allows us to take what this text has to offer in its own right. Having read, contemplated, and worked with this material as well as case studies and discussions about it that have been produced in Chinese publications, I can attest to its worth. Now that a groundbreaking and precise English translation and commentary have been published, I am sure many practitioners will put these ideas and formulas to use. I look forward to creating and reading more writings and translations that illustrate how practitioners use these beautiful ideas and formulas.

Preface

The Importance of History

1

Introduction

THE *FǓXÍNGJUÉ* PRESENTS A RARE voice from a distant time and space. It reflects the attainment of humans who consciously cultivated the ability to tune in to the "celestial movements" and to the resonances between the macrocosm and the microcosms of the human body, the social realm, and the natural world. In other words, these were humans who took seriously their pivotal role in the middle between Heaven and Earth. Connecting with Heaven in their lofty pursuit of immortality, they nevertheless recognized the need, in their human bodies, to keep their feet firmly planted on Earth. As such, they crafted the formulas and the herbal classification system found in this text so as to "provide assistance in the cultivation of Perfection, and to bring people back from the precipice of grave danger" by supplementing and draining each of the five *zàng* organs on the basis of differential diagnosis. In the words of the text itself:

今檢錄常情需用者六十首，備山中預防災疾之用耳。
檢用諸藥之要者，可默契經方之旨焉。經云：
在天成象，在地成形，

At present, here is a collection of sixty often-used formulas, to be ready for use in the mountains as a precaution against natural calamities and illness. As we examine the essence of how the various medicinals are used, we can form an invisible bond with the aim of the classical formulas through them. As the Classic states, 'in Heaven to complete the archetype, on earth to complete the form.'

To introduce you to the book you are holding in your hands, let me take you on two intertwined journeys: One, my personal journey in how this book came into existence, and two, the journey of the information in this book. With the help of that information, I hope you can appreciate the following translation for what it is and take from it the therapeutic and diagnostic advice, clinical inspiration, cultural and historical knowledge, or celestial perspective.

Starting with my own journey, it was maybe a dozen years ago that I first began to hear colleagues who practice Chinese medicine in what has become known as the "classical" tradition mention a text called the *Tāngyèjīng* 湯液經 ("Classic of Decoction"). According to their admittedly patchy historical knowledge, this was an important ancient classic that had been rediscovered recently and proven to be the ancestor of Zhāng Zhòngjǐng's 張仲景 work. It was also associated with a mythical figure named Yī Yǐn 伊尹, a mythological figure who rose from kitchen slave to minister at the Shāng court in the second millennium BCE. None of my clinical friends were able to give me a Chinese textual reference or cite a written source for these "*Tāngyèjīng* formulas," associated theories, and its classification scheme of twenty-five herbal substances into a five-times-five subcategorization based on the *wǔxíng* 五行 "five agents," a.k.a.

"five elements" or "five phases." Some colleagues had learned a whole "*Tāngyèjīng* system" of classifying individual herbal substances and organizing formulas in accordance with the *wǔxíng*. This "*Tāngyèjīng* system" was sometimes credited with providing the theoretical foundation for Zhāng Zhòngjǐng's classical formulas and, as such, was claimed to be foundational and essential to any *jīngfāng* ("classical formulas") approach to practicing traditional Chinese medicine.

Another angle from which I encountered this mysterious "*Tāngyèjīng*" was the group of the six spirit and two Yīn and Yáng "dawning" formulas that were also supposedly a part of this ancient classic. These were often cited as proof for the ancient date of the text, since they are clearly written in the "classical" style. When asked to elaborate on what they mean by this "classical" style, the advocates of the "*Tāngyèjīng* system" emphasize the affinity or even identity of this group of formulas with Zhāng Zhòngjǐng's formulas. And since their source, namely the so-called *Tāngyèjīng*, was an ancient "classic" (經 *jīng*), the argument went, it had to be ancestral to Zhāng Zhòngjǐng's own work, which was a mere "discussion" or "treatise" (論 *lùn*) and therefore a derivative from the canonical texts of the Hàn dynasty. This all sounded enticing, but my search for the *Tāngyèjīng* as a Hàn period or earlier classic only led to the occasional reference to a long-lost text of mythological origin.

In spite of this lack of information, as a former professor at a Chinese medicine college and somebody intimately involved with Chinese medicine education, I could see how this "*Tāngyèjīng*" information, especially the innovative view of medicinal substances through the lens of flavor could help students to appreciate the formula ingredients of traditional Chinese medicine as individual substances on their own terms. In fact, I view the in-depth teaching of classical formulas and their architecture as an important and promising advancement in what we usually call "herbal medicine" (even though it includes animal and mineral substances) in the West. The transmission of the *jīngfāng* ("classical formulas") style of practicing Chinese medicine is a long overdue development of Chinese medicine as practiced globally outside of China. The new level of education in and access to knowledge of "herbal medicine" in general, and the *jīngfāng* tradition in particular, has allowed an ever-increasing number of Western clinical practitioners of Chinese medicine to craft elegant and powerful individually tailored prescriptions and modifications. Obviously, such treatments, which we have all witnessed our senior Chinese colleagues and teachers apply, tend to be much more effective than crudely matching a limited number of syndromes to a limited number of formulas. As a result, the growing popularity of a "classical Chinese medicine" based on medicinal treatments, as has been practiced in China for roughly two millennia, has had a considerable positive impact on the practice of Chinese medicine in the West.

For these reasons, I always kept an eye out for information about this text. Being trained as a medical historian and translator specializing in early, classical, and medieval Chinese medical literature, I pride myself on my familiarity with this body of texts. While I cannot claim to have read every one of the texts written during this period cover to cover, I know the authors, titles, editions, and problems in the transmission of these texts, since they are, after all, limited in number. In this list of information sources that I constantly draw on in my own research, I do include archaeological discoveries of the last few decades, as well as textual sources from outside of China, such as the tenth-century Japanese compendium *Ishimpō* 醫心方 ("Formulas from the Heart of Medicine"), which consists of a marvelous collection of early medieval Chinese texts, of which many have not been preserved in China proper.

In this context, the single most important source of medical manuscripts to revolutionize our reading of the transmitted texts and revise our understanding of the history of Chinese medicine is the enormous treasure trove of texts that was discovered in the early 1900s in the so-called "library cave" in the Western desert outpost of Dūnhuáng (see below for more on this topic). In combination with the *Ishimpō*, this collection, made easily available in printed critical editions of great editorial quality, was already a key source of information for my doctoral research in the 1990s. It allowed me to pinpoint several changes introduced to the topic of my doctoral dissertation, Sūn Sīmiǎo's gynecological writings, by the Sòng dynasty editors of the text. Similarly, my doctoral advisor, Professor Donald Harper, was the author of the first and only English translation of the Mǎwángduī medical manuscripts, from a tomb closed in 168 BCE, which he published in 1998 as *Early Chinese Medical Literature: The Mawangdui Medical Manuscripts*. This publication forced medical historians to revise their theories about the origin and development of acupuncture and channel theory and also proved instrumental in dating different layers of the *Huángdì nèijīng*, for example. Thus, I am well familiar with the importance of archaeological discoveries and their potential to challenge, transform, and expand our previously existing knowledge on medical history. As an academic trained in the post-modern era, I am also keenly aware of the pitfalls of a closed mind when it comes to any aspect of history.

And yet, when I looked in my Chinese textbooks on medical history, in my collections of early and medieval text titles, and in the writings of major historical clinicians for traces of a so-called "Classic of Decoctions," whether as the literary ancestor of Zhāng Zhòngjǐng's work or just in general, I drew either blanks or the faintest references to a long-lost text of that title. What was going on here? Part of the problem was that the clinical colleagues who were sharing the content of this so-called *Tāngyèjīng* with me were not trained historians or philologians and did not have access to any original Chinese sources. They had acquired their information either second or third hand, or in exclusive classes not open to the public or professional feedback.

While costly private seminars in small closed groups is a teaching style popular in Western continuing education courses on Chinese medicine, it is unfortunately a mode of transmission that can allow for a dangerous absence of professional accountability and critical discussion among colleagues. Compounding this issue, instructors sometimes present passages from the classics in cherry-picked quotations and questionable interpretations out of context, on PowerPoint slides or in hand-outs that are not to be shared with outside experts, without contextualizing the presented information in the framework of peer-reviewed publications and the larger academic consensus. As a result, such presentations run the risk of disembodying historical literature and can end up serving to support a teacher's personal opinion rather than presenting a text authentically. This can leave students with a confused or even erroneous understanding of Chinese medical history.

In my quest for the origin of this "*Tāngyèjīng*," eventually I found an answer in a short article by Wang Shumin titled "Tangye jingfa: *a lost text in the* Hanshu *bibliography*," published in Vivienne Lo and Christopher Cullen, eds., *Medieval Chinese Medicine: The Dunhuang Medical Manuscripts* (see below for more on this article). As this contribution suggested, it was a text called *Fǔxíngjué zàngfǔ yòngyào fǎyào* 《輔行訣臟腑用藥法要》 ("Secret Tips for Helpful Action: The Key to Using Medicinals on the *Zàngfǔ* Organs," below abbreviated as *Fǔxíngjué*), believed to be a sixth- to tenth-century manuscript from the Dūnhuáng corpus of medical literature, that contained traces of this mysterious "Classical Methods of Decoctions." Bingo! I was happy to realize that this *Fǔxíngjué* was indeed a text that I had easy access to in several Chinese collections of Dūnhuáng medical literature in high-quality critical editions, sitting right there in my small personal library. So I went to work translating that text and then deciphering its long and convoluted textual history and relationship to this mysterious "Classic of Decoctions," which I have recorded for you in the following pages. While some of the figures and places below are of questionable relevance to factual history, I have included all the pieces that make up the puzzle of how this text has come to be discussed, taught, treated, and transmitted in China and abroad.

It really does make for a great story, and I hope that one of my readers will turn it into a movie production that I get to star in as Queen Mother of the West (since there are remarkably few female roles to be had here). Given the length of the journey of roughly four millennia and vast distances that we have to travel, I invite you to join me on a ride on the Chinese History Train with a comfortable window seat and occasional stops to catch fresh air and enjoy the local scenery. Do pack some good snacks! After we have visited all the major historical players, real and imagined, in Chapter Two of this Introduction, and looked at its global transmission in Chapter Three, we shall reconvene for a detailed analysis of the text's language and content in Chapter Four and take a cursory look at the different manuscript versions of the text in Chapter Five. I ask that readers who do not enjoy historical train rides and just don't have the patience for the admittedly very nerdy academic details in the following pages at least leaf through these sections and join the rest of us for the brief Conclusion in Chapter Six.

2

Textual History of the *Fǔxíngjué*: A Grand Plot

The history, interpretation, and past and present use of the *Fǔxíngjué zàngfǔ yòngyào fǎyào* 《輔行訣臟腑用藥法要》 ("Secret Tips for Helpful Action: The Key to Using Medicinals on the *Zàngfǔ* Organs") is a fascinating story spanning several millennia, countless dynasties, colorful figures of many social classes and professions, and vast geographical distances. And like a game of telephone, the eventual information that has arrived at our current final destination in my little writing studio in the woods of Whidbey Island in the Pacific Northwest may no longer have much in common with the original message. To entice the less historically inclined reader to grab a cup of tea, put up their feet, and take the time to read the following information, our Chinese History Train shall start with a juicy story of mythological dimensions.

2.1 Cook Yī Yǐn in the Shāng dynasty

Try to picture the most mysterious player in our drama: Yī Yǐn 伊尹, said to have been born in 1649 BCE, who left his mark on history as an ambitious kitchen slave. Brought to the Shāng court as part of a dowry gift, he so impressed the Shāng ruler Tāng with his insights, likely shared while serving him soup, that the king freed and eventually elevated him to the position of chancellor. In this position, Yī helped Tāng defeat the corrupt and declining Xià dynasty and establish the Shāng dynasty. He is said to have lived to a full hundred years of age, passing in 1549 BCE after having served under five successive Shāng kings.

In one version of early Chinese history, Yī Yǐn at one point usurped the throne, forced the fourth Shāng king Tài Jiǎ 太甲 into exile, and ruled illegitimately for 7 years before being deposed and killed by Tài Jiǎ upon the latter's return as the rightful heir. Other versions recount how Yī Yǐn the model minister virtuously coaxed the incapable and useless heir Tài Jiǎ into abdicating the throne and living in exile while Yī Yǐn reigned in his stead for several years, before passing the power back to a repentant and transformed king ready to resume his rightful place. According to the written record from the oracle bones, we do know that Yī Yǐn was honored throughout the Shāng dynasty as a key ancestral figure, receiving the same number of sacrificial cows as the Shāng ancestors themselves!

While the above makes for a great story, the written records on Yī Yǐn, whether oracle bones or bronzes or transmitted historical biographies compiled many many centuries later, fail us in mentioning anything at all concerning his involvement with medicine, formula literature, soups, or specifically with a text called the "Classic of Decoctions" 湯液經 *tāngyèjīng* or "Classical Methods of Decoctions" 湯液經法 *tāngyè jīngfǎ*. With two notable exceptions, it is not until the Sòng dynasty, two-and-a-half millennia later in the eleventh century CE, that authors begin routinely associating the illustrious minister Yī Yǐn with anything but exemplary government service.

2.2 The Catalogue of the Imperial Hàn Library

Our next stop on the Chinese History Train is not until about seventeen centuries later in the late Hàn dynasty, with a brief but, in the eyes of some proponents, significant line in the *Yìwénzhì* 藝文志 ("Treatise on Literature"), the bibliographical catalogue of the imperial Hàn library, composed in the early second century CE. The list of medical "classics and formulas" (*jīngfāng* 經方) in this text includes a mere reference to "classical methods of decoctions, 32 scrolls" (湯液經法三十二卷), with no named author or any additional information, sandwiched between "formulas for women and children, 19 scrolls" and "dietary taboos by Shénnóng and Huángdì, seven scrolls." Importantly, Yī Yǐn is not mentioned in this record at all. And perhaps even more importantly, when we read this line in the context of the *Yìwénzhì*, it may not even be referring to an actual text title that is 32 scrolls long, but more likely simply to 32 scrolls that contain "methods from the classics for [preparing] decoctions." As such, we cannot use this short phrase as our sole historical evidence for the existence of a text of this title in the Hàn dynasty.

2.3 Huángfǔ Mì's "A-Z Classic of Acupuncture and Moxibustion"

Our next stop is less than a hundred years later: In his preface to the *Zhēnjiǔ jiǎyǐjīng* 針灸甲乙經 ("A–Z Classic of Acupuncture and Moxibustion"), the medical author Huángfǔ Mì (215–282 CE) gives us a crash course in medical history. After describing how the Divine Farmer Shénnóng tasted a hundred herbs and the Yellow Emperor Huángdì interviewed his various medical advisors to perfect his "Dào of needling," we find the following sentence:

伊尹以亞聖之才，撰用神農本草以為湯液。

Yī Yǐn used his talent of a lesser sage and picked up the Divine Farmer's materia medica to make his decoctions.

For full disclosure, I should mention that many modern interpreters of this passage whose intention it is to prove the historicity of the *Tāngyèjīng* as an ancient text authored by Yī Yǐn, whether Chinese or Western, choose to read 神農本草 ("Divine Farmer's materia medica") and 湯液 ("decoctions") as text titles and format or translate them as such in this context. In my eyes, this is an interpretation that falsifies the original meaning of the text. In my experience with classical literature, had Huángfǔ Mì truly wanted to say "Divine Farmer's Classic of Materia Medica" and "Classic of Decoctions," he would have added the simple character 經 *jīng* ("classic") in each case. What I have given you is a very straightforward, literal translation. In fact, even translating 神農本草 as "Divine Farmer's materia medica" is a bit of an interpretation, since literally the phrase just says "Divine Farmer's roots and herbs." The commonly used standard abbreviation of the full text title *Shénnóng běncǎojīng* 神農本草經 ("Divine Farmer's Classic of Materia Medica") has never been *Shénnóng běncǎo* ("Shénnóng's materia medica) but always *Běnjīng* 本經 ("Root Classic"), a term that clearly refers to a text, while "Shénnóng's materia medica" merely refers to the medicinal substances employed or studied by Shénnóng.

After Huángfǔ Mì next mentions a string of famous Warring States and Hàn dynasty physicians, he emphasizes the work of Huà Tuó 華佗 and Zhāng Zhòngjǐng 張仲景 in particular as having "marvelous formulas and extraordinary treatments" and describes their medical feats. Then there is our second piece of evidence:

仲景論廣伊尹湯液為數十卷，用之多驗。

[Zhāng] Zhòngjǐng discussed and expanded Yī Yǐn's decoctions to create several tens of scrolls. When you use these, they are mostly effective.

And that is the full extent of Huángfǔ Mì's description of Zhāng Zhòngjǐng's involvement with Yī Yǐn's decoctions. He then continues his account with Wáng Shūhé and discusses the composition of the *Huángdì nèijīng* 黃帝內經 ("Yellow Emperor's Inner Classic") in 18 scrolls as a combination of the *Sùwèn* 素問 ("Plain Questions") and

Zhēnjīng 針經 ("Needle Classic," the text we now know as *Língshū* 靈樞 "Divine Pivot") with nine scrolls each. As you may be able to see from this brief account, it is obvious in all of these other passages when Huángfǔ is talking about a text, as opposed to describing a person and their activity.

In other words, and to conclude this section, these two statements cannot be taken as proof that Zhāng Zhòngjǐng actually based his entire *Shānghánlùn* 傷寒論 ("Discussion on Cold Damage") on a text called *Tāngyè jīngfǎ* 《湯液經法》 authored by Yī Yǐn, nor that Huángfǔ Mì had access to such a text or even to such rudimentary information as the number of scrolls, which he surely would have included. When Sòng period medical commentators like Lín Yì 林億 expand on these two phrases almost a thousand years later, such statements again cannot be taken as proof for the existence of this text or for Zhāng Zhòngjǐng's reliance on it in crafting his own famous formula collection. Lín Yì, after all, was much more careful in his words than many modern teachers and merely stated without any reference to a *jīng* "classic" that "Zhòngjǐng based [his work] on Yī Yǐn's methods" 「仲景本伊尹之法」.

2.4 Zhāng Zhòngjǐng and the "Discussion on Cold Damage"

For more information on the role of a lost text called *Tāngyè jīngfǎ* as a potential influence on Zhāng Zhòngjǐng's work, we actually have to put the History Train in reverse for a moment since we appear to have rolled right by the great Master of Cold Damage himself, who lived ca. 150–219 CE. And that omission of a stop has actually been intentional, and needs to be emphasized as such, since the nature of this argument is precisely the striking absence of this title from the list of sources Zhāng Zhòngjǐng himself provided us with in his preface! Here are his own words:

余宗族素多，向余二百，建安紀年以來，猶未十稔，其死亡者，三分有二，傷寒十居其七。感往昔之淪喪，傷橫夭之莫救，乃勤求古訓，博采眾方，撰用素問、九卷、八十一難、陰陽大論、胎臚藥錄，並平脈辨証，為傷寒雜病論合十六卷。雖未能盡愈諸病，庶可以見病知源。若能尋余所集，思過半矣。

My ancestral clan has always been numerous, with more than two hundred members in the past. But since the first year of Jiàn'ān (i.e., 196 CE), in less than ten years, the proportion of those who have perished has been two out of three, with cold damage claiming seven out of ten of these. Deeply affected by this ruinous loss in my past and by the failure to rescue them from damage and premature death, I have diligently sought out the ancient instructions and collected a great number of formulas far and wide. I have chosen the Sùwèn, *the* Língshū, *the* Nànjīng, *the* Yīnyáng dàlùn, *the* Tāilú yàolù, *and the* Píngmài biànzhèng,[1] *to compose the* Shānghán zábìng lùn *in sixteen scrolls. Even though you will not yet be able to exhaustively cure all the various diseases, you may be able to look at a disease and know its origin. If you can unravel what I have collected here, you will have thought through more than half [of all problems you might face].*

After a brief rumination on the profound subtleties of Yīn and Yáng and their medical applications, Zhāng continues by presenting us with a list of the famous medical figures up to his times:

[1] The last two sources mentioned are titles of medical texts that are now lost. *Yīnyáng dàlùn* may refer to a lost text or quite possibly to chapter five of the *Sùwèn,* which is titled *Yīnyáng yìngxiàng dàlùn* 陰陽應象大論 ("Great Discourse on the Resonant Manifestations of Yīn and Yáng"). Also, the discerning reader may notice that I have taken the liberty of translating the Chinese 九卷 (lit. "Nine Scrolls") into *Língshū* and 八十一難 (lit. "81 Difficulties") into *Nànjīng*. This was not done lightly and I am simply following the academic consensus.

上古有神農、黃帝、岐伯、伯高、雷公、少俞、少師、
仲文。中世有長桑、扁鵲。漢有公乘陽慶及倉公。
下此以往，未之聞也。

In the ancient past there were Shénnóng, Huángdì, Qí Bó, Bó Gāo, Léi Gōng, Shào Yú, Shào Shā, and Zhòng Wén. In mid-antiquity there were Cháng Sāng and Biǎn Què. During the Hàn dynasty, there were Gōng Shèn Yáng Qìng and Cāng Gōng. After these, I have not heard of anybody else.

Given the comprehensive nature of these two lists of famous texts and doctors, it is highly significant that neither Yī Yǐn nor a "Classic of Decoctions" or "Classical Methods of Decoctions" are mentioned at all. It is well-known that traditional Chinese medical authors, unlike their Western counterparts until quite recently, tend to emphasize the ancient sources of their work, whether in commentaries and discussions or in prefaces and introductions. I simply cannot think of a reason why Zhāng Zhòngjǐng would have failed to mention Yī Yǐn's formula collection if he had been aware of, had access to, and made use of, such an important and groundbreaking "classic." In my mind, the glaring absence of this title and its author here is one of the most convincing arguments against this notion that a mythological *Tāngyèjīng* by Yī Yǐn was a key source for Zhāng Zhòngjǐng's own formula collection. And this big historical question mark does not even address the problem of the relationship between that text and our source text, the *Fǔxíngjué* , which we shall turn to next.

2.5 Táo Hóngjǐng's Cauldrons of Immortality (fifth–sixth century)

After a nice cup of tea in the dining car of our History Train to help us speed past a few centuries, we arrive at our next stop in the early sixth century, high up into the remote crags and crevices of Mount Máo 茅山, a celebrated sacred Daoist mountain in China's Southeast. Here we meet up with the alleged author of the *Fǔxíngjué*, a colorful Daoist figure named Táo Hóngjǐng 陶弘景 who is known in Chinese history primarily as the founder of Máoshān Daoism. Slowly we are starting to stand on slightly more solid ground, academically speaking, since Táo is listed in the front of the *Fǔxíngjué* itself as its "compiler":

梁華陽隱居陶弘景撰

Compiled by Táo Hóngjǐng, hermit from Huáyáng, during the Liáng dynasty

If we read this subtitle as a factual statement, it raises all sorts of questions: What exactly was Táo Hóngjǐng's role in the composition of this text? Was he the creator of this entire text, the compiler of different texts, or merely the editor of a single source, to which he only added the occasional comment? In other words, what did his source text or texts look like, if there were any, before and after his involvement? And, to open a whole other can of worms, what are the differences between Táo's work, if it ever even existed, and the text transmitted to us in more than twenty different manuscript versions today?

As a conscientious academic and critical thinker, however, I must first emphasize that we can never take a Chinese text's purported authorship at face value. Especially in the absence of any other supporting evidence, it is quite reasonable to assume that Táo's name only came to be attached to this text retroactively and that the creator of the text merely added Táo's name to the text to give it an air of antiquity and authority. Just as some modern proponents like to claim that the *Tāngyèjīng* was composed by Yī Yǐn in the ancient Shāng dynasty or as modern pharmacies in both China and the West sell "ancient Chinese secrets," there was nothing to stop a good writer in traditional China from adding Táo as the author or compiler of the *Fǔxíngjué*! In fact, one of the strongest arguments against Táo Hóngjǐng's direct involvement with the *Fǔxíngjué* is the fact that he is not mentioned anywhere else throughout history as the author or compiler of this text, or even in any way associated with either the *Tāngyèjīng* or the *Fǔxíngjué*.

Táo Hóngjǐng was certainly an illustrious and highly esteemed figure in early medieval history. Thus we know quite a bit of detail about his life, including the precise dates of his birth and death, namely 456 and 536 CE.[2] Of course he is most famous for compiling the *Shénnóng běncǎojīng jízhù* 神農本草經輯注 ("Collected Commentaries on the Divine Farmer's Classic of Materia Medica," ca. 500 CE). In the preface of that work, he does mention a number of texts and doctors from the second through fifth centuries beyond the Divine Farmer as his sources of information: Zhāng Zhòngjǐng, Huà Tuó 華佗, the *Tóngjūn cǎiyào lù* 桐君採藥錄 ("Master Tóng's records of picking medicinals"), the *Yàoduì* 藥對 ("Comparison of medicinals"), and the doctors Wú Pǔ 吳普 and Lǐ Dāngzhī 李當之. He further states that he has gathered them all together to inform his revision of the *Shénnóng běncǎojīng*. While the *Fǔxíngjué* is obviously primarily a formula text, the central and, to many contemporary practitioners, most innovative and fascinating, textual layer concerns what is in my translation Section Four on "The Five Flavors and Twenty-Five Medicinals." This section is a statement about materia medica and their categorization into a five-fold structure based on the *wǔxíng*. If Táo had had access to this information on categorizing materia medica when he compiled his famous commentary *Shénnóng*

[2] See my biography of Táo Hóngjǐng in W.F. and Helen Bynum, eds., *Dictionary of Medical Biography* (Greenwood Press, 2006).

běncǎojīng jízhù 神農本草經輯注, I cannot imagine that it would not have influenced that work, or at least been mentioned by him!

Táo's two other surviving works are foundational scriptures in the esteemed tradition of Shàngqīng Daoism: *Zhēn'gào* 真誥 ("Declarations of the Perfected Ones," ca. 492 CE) and *Dēngzhēn yǐnjué* 登真隱訣 ("Hidden Instructions for the Ascent to Perfection," before 500 CE). In addition to his philological and alchemical studies and his life-long spiritual practices in the pursuit of longevity and immortality, he tutored imperial princes and commanded a section of the palace guards. After an active politically engaged life, he retired in 492 to withdraw as a hermit to the mountains, where he established and presided over a monastic community of Daoist adepts, even protecting them from political persecution due to his close friendship with powerful figures like the Buddhist emperor Wǔ of the Liáng dynasty 梁武帝. In addition to these three surviving texts, he is recorded as the author of several other texts that have been lost, including a book of family recipes, a collection of eye formulas, another comprehensive text on medicinals, and a collection of emergency formulas called "101 Formulas to Keep Up Your Sleeve." We know about these texts from the many prefaces that have been written to various editions of his extant books and from bibliographic catalogues of the Suí and Táng dynasties. It strikes me as inconceivable that such an influential person would have compiled this important innovative text without such a feat leaving any trace until the text reappeared in a doctor's recollection of a manuscript purchased by his grandfather and destroyed soon afterwards almost 1500 years later!

Moreover, if we are to take Táo Hóngjǐng's own work as evidence, his edition of the "Divine Farmer's Classic of Materia Medica" stands out for faithfully distinguishing between the original source text and his various additions, which are marked in different-colored ink and identified as commentary by himself or "illustrious physicians" (名醫 *míngyī*). By contrast, the *Fǔxíngjué* contains multiple layers of written and even graphic information, with no comments on where these layers come from, except for the occasional reference to a "classic" and to a handful of notes by "the recluse Táo." And whenever the text does mention a "classic," it is usually a reference to a citation from the *Nèijīng* (see more on citations in the *Fǔxíngjué* itself in the following section).

On the other hand, if we take the story of the transmission of this text at face value, the text must have been so important that it was carefully preserved for several centuries, even though it never appeared in the imperial catalogues of library holdings, lists of sources by medical authors like Cháo Yuánfāng 巢元方 or Sūn Sīmiǎo 孫思邈, records of Táo's many disciples and followers, or collections of medieval medical sources like the *Ishimpō* 醫心方 ("formulas from the heart of medicine"). Moreover, after supposedly being carried over a distance of almost three thousand kilometers to a remote Western outpost in the desert, it was eventually sealed as one of the precious gifts of humanity in the Mògāo 莫高 caves, only to show up again a thousand years later in a copied manuscript submitted to the China Academy of Chinese Medicine in Běijīng in the 1970s.

As the inclusion of the *Fǔxíngjué* in multiple collections of Dūnhuáng 敦煌 medical manuscripts shows, it is the current academic consensus in China that the copy submitted to the China Academy most likely represents not a modern forgery but a medieval text of historical significance. As such, but only as such, it carries great value for the history of medicine and fills an important gap in our understanding of the development of formula literature. Any historical claims beyond that, however, do not hold up, regardless of the clinical value of the text in and of itself. But let us not jump ahead, but instead spend a little while in the delightful crisp mountain air of Mount Máo, before getting back into our stuffy train compartment. Let us finally unscroll the *Fǔxíngjué* itself to look for hints of Táo's, or his impersonator's, role and a possible relationship to Yī Yǐn's *Tāngyè jīng[fǎ]* in the formation of the text.

2.6 Possible References to the *Tāngyèjīng* in the *Fǔxíngjué*

First, as already alluded to in the discussion of Huángfǔ Mì's mention of Yī Yǐn's decoctions above, in classical Chinese medical literature 湯液 *tāngyè* is a fairly common expression that simply means "decoction/s," while 經 *jīng* means "classic/-al"[3] and 經法 *jīngfǎ* and 經方 *jīngfāng* are also fairly common phrases meaning "classical methods" and "classical formulas," respectively. All of these phrases are found throughout the received classical medical literature and do not once refer to the *Tāngyèjīng* 湯液經 ("Decoctions Classic") as the title of a text![4] We must therefore never read these phrases as necessarily or automatically referring to the title of an obscure text whose very existence is debatable. Unless there is clear evidence that they are referring to an actual text title in a particular context, they cannot be interpreted or "translated" as "*Tāngyèjīng* methods/formulas," especially when the text only mentions a partial

[3] The meaning of "classic/-al" or "canon/-ical" is in addition to the other meanings of the character 經: "warp," "channel/conduit," "constant," and even "menstrual period."

[4] Searching the phrase 「湯液」 *tāngyè* "decoctions" in the *Nèijīng* resulted in ten hits, none of which referred to a "*Tāngyèjīng*" as a text title, but all of which simply meant "decoctions." See https://ctext.org/huangdi-neijing/zh?searchu=%E6%B9%AF%E6%B6%B2. Similarly, searching 「湯液」 in the *Bèijí qiānjīn yàofāng* 備急千金要方 resulted in four hits, each meaning "decoctions" and not once referring to the *Tāngyèjīng* either (https://ctext.org/wiki.pl?if=gb&res=236578&searchu=%E6%B9%AF%E6%B6%B2). A search for 「經方」 *jīngfāng* resulted in eight hits in the *Bèijí qiānjīn yàofāng*, all just with the standard meaning "classical formulas."

phrase like 「湯液」 *tāngyè* ("decoctions") or 「經方」 *jīngfāng* ("classical formulas").

Having any of these phrases enclosed in modern Chinese publications in 《such brackets as these》 to designate them as a book title is a modern practice and therefore obviously only occurs in modern editions of historical literature. It is actually an interpretation of a historical text that is added by a modern editor and must therefore always be treated with caution. This is especially true when these are found in publications that are not produced or curated by renowned medical historians but by clinicians with inadequate training to produce historically accurate critical editions. Finding these brackets in modern editions thus cannot be a valid argument that these terms, in that specific context, refer to the text. Similarly, it is ahistorical and misleading for so-called "translations" of the *Fǔxíngjué* in Western languages to then leave these phrases untranslated in Pīnyīn or mark them otherwise as the title of the book "*Tāngyèjīng*," instead of translating them as "decoction" and "classical...."

After many years of reading, translating, and teaching traditional Chinese medical literature and classical Chinese language, I have arrived at the conclusion that classical Chinese can and will be as precise as the author needed or intended it to be. So when a classical author wanted to clearly express to a reader that they were talking about a book title or citing a text, even if only as a paraphrase, there were many ways to do so: Most notably, and as is done many times in the *Fǔxíngjué* itself to refer to quotations from other classics, the character 云 *yūn* ("... states/says:...") is employed as the classical equivalent of modern quotation marks. Alternatively, a classical writer either spells out the full title of a text, combines it with the author's name, or employs such an obvious abbreviation of the title that it could not be read as anything else, such as the abbreviation 本經 *běnjīng* ("root classic") that is used consistently to refer to the

Shénnóng běncǎo jīng《神農本草經》("Divine Farmer's Classic of Materia Medica").

With that settled, let us take a closer look at occurrences of any of these terms in the *Fǔxíngjué* itself, since these are always cited as the main proof for reading this entire text as a faithful early medieval copy of a much earlier *Tāngyéjīng* and therefore as quintessentially a Hàn dynasty text.

2.7 Occurrences of the terms 經 *jīng* ("classic" or "classical"), 湯液 *tāngyè* ("decoctions"), and 伊尹 Yī Yǐn in the *Fǔxíngjué*

To begin with, the text uses the term 經 *jīng* "classic/classical" in the following contexts and meanings, which I have highlighted in each passage: First and in most instances, it functions as an abbreviated reference to the *Nèijīng*《內經》("Inner Classic," i.e., the *Huángdì nèijīng* 黃帝內經 "Yellow Emperor's Inner Classic"). For example, here is the first instance of this use from Section 1.2, where it refers to *Sùwèn* 素問 ("Plain Questions," i.e. the first half of the *Nèijīng*), Chapter Twenty-Two.

> 陶云：肝德在散。故經云以辛補之，以酸瀉之。肝苦急，急食甘以緩之。適其性而衰也。
>
> *Táo [Hóngjǐng] states: The special power of the liver lies in dispersing. Therefore the Classic says to use the acrid flavor to supplement it and to use the sour flavor to drain it. When the liver suffers from tension, urgently consume sweet substances to slacken it. This is a case of weakening it by conforming to its nature.*

In the next instance, Section 1.3, it is used first in the meaning of "channel" but then in the following sentence again as a reference to *Língshū* 71:

取其經手少陰、太陽，及舌下血者。其變，刺郗中血者。邪在心，則病心中痛，善悲，時眩仆，視有餘不足而調之。經云：諸邪在心者，皆心胞代受。。。

Choose its channels, the Hand Shàoyīn and Tàiyáng, and draw blood below the tongue. ...

The presence of evil in the heart results in suffering from pain in the center of the heart, a tendency to grief, and periodic dizziness and falling over. See whether there is excess or insufficiency, and attune it accordingly. The Classic states: For the various sorts of evil in the Qì, the pericardium always contracts them instead...

The passages on the other *zàng* organs in the first section similarly contain the phrase 「經云」 ("the Classic states") to refer to famous passages from the *Nèijīng*.

The next three occurrences of the character 經 *jīng* are found in the introductory essay attributed to Táo in Section Three, the "five formulas for supplementing the five *zàng* organs." I am quoting the passage in its entirety so that the critical reader can form their own opinion by looking at the use of the characters in context.

陶云：經方有救諸勞損病方，亦有五首。然綜觀其要義，蓋不外虛候方加減而已。錄出以備修真之輔，拯人之危也。

然其方意深妙，非俗淺所識，緣諸損候，藏氣互乘，虛實雜錯，藥味寒熱並行，補瀉相參，先聖遺奥，出人意表。

漢晉以還，諸名醫輩，張機、衛汜［汎］、華元化、吳普、皇甫玄晏、支法師、葛稚川、范將軍等，皆當代名賢，咸師式此湯液經法，愍救疾苦，造福含靈。其間增減，雖各擅其異，或致新效，似亂舊經，而其旨趣，仍方圓之規矩也。

Táo [Hōngjǐng] states: Among the classical formulas, there are the those that rescue from the various illnesses of taxation injury, and there are also five of them. This being so, when we look at the key principle underlying all of them, they are merely modifications of formulas for vacuity signs, and nothing more. I have written them out to provide assistance in the cultivation of Perfection, and to bring people back from the precipice of grave danger.

And yet, the meaning of these formulas is profound and subtle, and hence not something that shallow minds can comprehend. Following along with the various signs of injury, the zàng *organs' Qì exploit each other, vacuity and repletion become intermixed, among the medicinal flavors hot and cold act simultaneously, and supplementing and draining join hands. The relics left behind by the sages from the past are enigmatic and go far beyond the superficial limitations of what people are able to project into the future.*

Ever since the Hàn and Jìn dynasties, the various famous physicians, Zhāng Jī, Wèi Xùn, Huà Tuó, Wú Pǔ, Huángfǔ Mì, Zhī Fǎcún, Gě Hóng, Fàn Wāng, etc., all the famous men of virtue of our times, every teacher has emulated these classical methods of decoctions to compassionately save people from illness and suffering and to bestow blessings on all sentient beings. Even though their modifications each excel in the differences that set them apart and may bring about new efficacy, seeming to revolutionize the old classics, yet their ultimate goal still lines up squarely with the old standards.

This is one of the key passages cited by proponents of reading the *Fǔxíngjué* as a medieval copy of an ancient formula text by Yī Yǐn called "Classic (or "Classical Methods) of Decoctions" 湯液經（法）*Tāngyè jīng[fǎ]*. Three things strike me as important to note: First, the absence of Yī Yǐn's name as the author of the text or his role in authoring it. Second, the absence of a clear reference to a single ancient text as a source for this compilation, with no reference to the transmission of such a text, to the shape of the supposed source, such as number of scrolls, essays, or formulas, or to the structure or content of the original text if there ever was one. Instead— and this is is my third point — Táo, or rather his impersonator, emphasizes the diversity of practices among the famous physicians of his age (from the late Hàn dynasty on) and their creativity in "revolutionizing the old classics." This statement here does not support, or even runs counter, to modern representations of Táo's role in the *Fǔxíngjué* as being limited to faithfully copying an existing ancient source, especially one with the status of a "classic," which is not a term used lightly in early Chinese literature. This is particularly relevant if we further try to claim that this same "classic" had already been the direct source of Zhāng Zhòngjǐng's writings in the late Hàn dynasty.

The next occurrence of the character 經 in the *Fǔxíngjué* is found in the concluding essay of this same chapter where the reference to the "Classic" again clearly refers to *Sùwèn* 22:

> 陶云：經云：毒藥攻邪，五菜為充，五果為助，五穀為養，五畜為益。爾乃大湯之設。今所錄者，皆小湯耳。若欲作大湯者，補肝湯內加羊肝，補心加雞心，補脾加牛肉，補肺加犬肺，補腎加豬腎，各一具，即成也。

> *Táo [Hóngjǐng] states: According to the Classic, toxic medicinals attack evils, the five vegetables provide fullness, the five fruits provide assistance, the five grains provide nourishment, and the five farm animals provide additional benefit. This then is how you build large decoctions.*

What is recorded in the present text are all small decoctions. if you want to turn them into large decoctions, add mutton liver to the decoction for supplementing the liver, chicken heart to supplement the heart, beef flesh to supplement the spleen, dog lung to supplement the lung, and pig kidney to supplement the kidney, 1 piece each, and that makes it complete.

Probably the single most important argument for reading the *Fǔxíngjué* as a copy of Yī Yǐn's "Decoction Classic" is found in the introductory essay to Section Four on the five flavors and twenty-five medicinals. Again, it is essential that we examine this essay in full here so that the critical reader can draw their own conclusions on the significance of this statement by the "hermit Táo":

陶隱居云：依神農本經及桐君採藥錄，上中下三品之藥，凡三百六十五味，以應周天之度，四時八節之氣。商有聖相伊尹，撰湯液經三卷，為方，亦三百六十首：上品上藥，為服食補益方者百二十者；中品中藥，為療疾祛邪之方，亦百十十首；下品毒藥，為殺蟲辟邪之方，亦百二十首。凡共三百六十首也。實萬代醫家之規範，蒼生護命之大寶也。

今檢錄常情需用者六十首，備山中預防災疾之用耳。檢用諸藥之要者，可默契經方之旨焉。經云：在天成象，在地成形，天有五氣，化生五味，五味之變，不可勝數。

Hermit Táo [Hóngjǐng] states: According to the Divine Farmer's Classic of Materia Medica *and* Lord Tóng's Record of Picking Medicinals, *the three grades of medicinals, — upper, middle, and lower — altogether comprise 365 substances, thereby resonating with the complete 360-degree circle of the universe and with the Qì of the Four Seasons and Eight Nodes. In the Shāng dynasty, there was the sagely minister Yī Yǐn who composed a* Classic of Decoctions *in three scrolls, consisting of formulas, also with 360 entries. The upper grade with the upper medicinals consisted of formulas for alchemical foods and supplementing and boosting, of which there were 120. The middle grade with middle medicinals consisted of formulas for curing illness and driving away evils, of which there were also 120. The lower grade with toxic medicinals consisted of formulas for killing worms and warding off evils, of which there were also 120. So in total there were altogether 360 entries. Truly, this has been the standard for myriad generations of physicians and the great treasure for protecting the life of all the people.*

At present, here is a collection of sixty often-used formulas, to be ready for use in the mountains as a precaution against natural calamities and illness. As we examine the essence of how the various medicinals are used, we can form an invisible bond with the aim of the classical formulas through them. As the classic states, in Heaven to complete the archetype, on earth to complete the form. Heaven has the Five Qì, which transform to engender the Five Flavors. The alterations of the Five Flavors are too many to count.

Let us take this essay apart and look closely at each instance of the use of 經 *jīng* "classic" found here. The first passage is obviously just a reference to the book title *Shénnóng běncǎojīng*, which we can skip over.

The second highlighted passage is the most interesting one. This is the only instance in the entire *Fǔxíngjué* where a comment attributed to Táo mentions Yī Yǐn and clearly refers to a text called the "Classic of Decoctions." The information that this ancient text consists of three scrolls and contains 360 formulas, divided into three grades and thereby following the structure of the *Shénnóng běncǎojīng* with its 360 medicinals, which are also arranged in three grades of directly parallel functions, is completely new and not replicated anywhere else in the received literature. As you might remember, Táo was instrumental in the transmission of the *Shénnóng běncǎojīng* by editing, rearranging, and commenting on it in what has become the standard edition to this day. The evaluation of the formulas attributed to Táo here, with the superior grade being used for alchemical transformation for the purpose of spiritual cultivation, longevity, and eventual immortality, and the inferior grade being associated with "toxic medicinals... for killing worms and warding off evils," is directly in line with Táo's evaluation of the medicinals in the *Shénnóng běncǎojīng* and reflects Táo's background as a dedicated practitioner of Daoist alchemical practices in pursuit of immortality.

As a side note, should it not also make us wonder that Táo does mention Yī Yǐn in the preface to his famous revision of the *Shénnóng běncǎojīng* but only as an ancient sage who "disseminated the Hundred Grains, bestowing their benevolence on all living people," without a word about his decoctions, much less about the famous formula collection attributed to him thousands of years later? Here is the passage in question from Táo's preface to the *Shénnóng běncǎojīng*:

> 舊說皆稱神農本草經，余以為信然。昔神農氏之王天下也，畫易卦以通鬼神之情；造耕種，以省煞害之弊；宣藥療疾，以拯夭傷之命。此三道者，歷群聖而滋彰。文王、孔子，彖象繇辭，幽贊人天。后稷、伊尹，播厥百谷，惠被生民。岐、皇、彭、扁，振揚輔導，恩流含氣。並歲逾三千，民到於今賴之。
>
> *The old explanations all refer to a* Divine Farmer's Classic of Materia Medica. *I consider this to be reliable. In the past, in his rule of Under Heaven, the Divine Farmer drew the trigrams of the* Classic of Changes *to provide access to the dispositions of the supernatural entities; set up the plowing and planting of fields to save people from death from terminal injuries; and promulgated [information on] medicinals and the curing of illnesses, to rescue from the fate of premature loss*

of life and damages. These three Teachings (lit. Dao) were [then] enriched and illuminated by passing through large numbers of sages. King Wén and Confucius added judgments, images, and commentaries, acclaiming humanity and heaven through obscurity. Hòu Jì and Yī Yǐn disseminated the Hundred Grains, bestowing their benevolence on all living people. Qí Bó, Huángdì, Péngzǔ, and Biǎn Què provided guidance and support with great fervor. In this way, the [Divine Farmer's] beneficence has circulated and remained alive. And even though three thousand years have gone by, the people still rely on it to this day!

Returning to the essay in the *Fǔxíngjué* quoted above, the third and fourth instances of using the character *jīng* in this important passage occur in the context of a generic reference to "classical formulas" and then once again to introduce a "statement from the Classic." In this case, the original source of this so-called "classic" appears to be the *Zhōu Yì Xìcí* 《周易繫辭》(Appendix on the Classic of Changes), one of the famous commentaries on the *Yìjīng* traditionally attributed to Confucius.

Proceeding with our analysis of the *Fǔxíngjué* for references to Yī Yǐn and his "Decoction Classic," the brief concluding statement at the end of Section Four includes the character 經 twice:

經云：主於補瀉者為君，數量同於君而非主故為臣，
從於佐監者為佐使。
陶隱居曰：此圖乃湯液經法盡要之妙，學者能
諳於此，醫道畢矣。

The Classic states: [Substances] that are in charge of supplementing and draining constitute the rulers; [substances] that are identical in quantity to the ruler but are not in charge constitute the ministers; [substances that] follow to assist the supervisors constitute the assistants and envoys.

The hermit Táo [Hóngjǐng] states: This chart indeed [reflects] the utterly significant subtlety of the classical methods of decoctions. When those who study them are able to know them by heart, their Dào of medicine has reached its destination!

Regarding the first instance, I have unfortunately been unable to trace this quotation from a "classic" back to a known textual source. As such, it is possible that we are in this case indeed dealing with a citation from the "Classic of Decoctions." But if this were the case, wouldn't the fact that this particular statement is identified specifically as a quotation from this classic imply that the rest of the text is not, especially since this reference to a "statement from a classic" is not found in the comments attributed to Táo but is formatted as part of the actual text that precedes those? In other words, this is the actual source text citing yet another source, so if the source text is supposed to be the *Tāngyèjīng*, it doesn't make sense that it would be quoting itself. At the same time, the language in this quotation is reminiscent of Táo's preface to the *Shénnóng běncǎojīng*, which twice classifies medicinals in the three grades of "rulers," "ministers," and "assistants and envoys." Given how loosely worded some of the other quotations of classics in the *Fǔxíngjué* are, it is possible that the *Shénnóng běncǎojīng* is the "classic" referred to here. Alternatively, it could refer to *Sùwèn* 74, another "classic" since it is part of the "Yellow Emperor's Inner Classic," which states:

主病之謂君，佐君之謂臣，應臣之謂使，
非上下三品之謂也。

[Substances] that rule disease are called ruler, those that support the ruler are called minister, and those that respond to the minister are called envoys. This is not a reference to the three grades of superiority and inferiority.

The second occurrence in the concluding note attributed to Táo is the only instance where the *Fǔxíngjué* actually refers to what could be read as the full title *Tāngyè jīngfǎ* 湯液經法 ("classical methods of decoctions"). It is just as possible, however, that this is a generic reference, as in the use of 經法 "classical methods" above, to the "classical methods" for composing and brewing "decoctions." There is simply not enough evidence here to draw a firm conclusion one way or the other, especially since we have no other independent reference to such a chart anywhere else in the received literature and that this note is only found on a manuscript dating to the late twentieth century. For more information on this chart specifically, see my discussion below.

The next and final use of the character 經 *jīng* in the *Fǔxíngjué* is found in the introduction to Section Five on the Classical Treatments for External Contraction:

> 弘景曰：外感天行，經方之治，有二旦、六神大小等湯。昔南陽張機，依此諸方，撰為《傷寒論》一部，療治明悉，後學咸尊奉之。
>
> 山林僻居，倉卒難防外感之疾，日數傳變，生死往往在三五日間，豈可疏忽。若能深明此數方者，則庶無蹈險之虞也。今亦錄而識之。

> *[Táo] Hóngjǐng states: Among the classical formula treatments for external contractions of celestial movements, there are the two Dawning and six Spirit decoctions, in major and minor grades. In the past Zhāng Jī from Nányáng relied on these various formulas to compose the* Treatise on Cold Damage *in one section. Given how incisive and comprehensive these treatments are, later students all revere them.*
>
> *Those of us who dwell secluded in mountains and forests are all of sudden confronted with critical illnesses of external contraction that*

are difficult to avoid. With numerous transmissions and changes each day, life and death are often on the line within only three to five days. How could we possibly be careless about this! If we are able to deeply understand these several formulas, then we might just avoid the worrisome prospect of this risk. At present I have also recorded them and committed them to memory.

This final section of the *Fǔxíngjué* poses an interesting challenge. Compared to the previous textual layers, and in light of this comment attributed to Táo here, these formulas do in fact seem to be more directly derived, or even literally copied, from an earlier, "classical" source. The close textual parallels to some of Zhāng Zhòngjǐng's formulas here do suggest that this last section of the *Fǔxíngjué* was either based on Zhāng Zhongjǐng's work or that the two texts shared a common source that has not been preserved anywhere else. Whether this shared source was in fact Yī Yǐn's "Classic of Decoctions" is impossible to ascertain and perhaps irrelevant. It should be noted that the comment attributed to Táo does not refer to such a text as the source here but merely refers to "classical formulas for external contractions of movements in the sky."

To be sure, the absence of any actual evidence to unequivocally support or contradict a thesis is always less convincing than a clear-cut finding. Nevertheless, when we now step back and look at all of these instances comprehensively, a picture emerges of the *Fǔxíngjué* as a medieval text consisting of multiple textual layers, with clearly identified, and verifiable, quotations from known classics, different and unrelated groups of formulas, and commentary from no earlier than the sixth century, but with no single passage or formula directly and unequivocally identifiable as a citation from a text called "Classic of Decoctions," whether by Yī Yǐn or by anybody else. Given the fact that even the supposed notes by Táo Hóngjǐng are of questionable historicity and are more likely to have come from Táo's followers or even from an impersonator several centuries later, the fact that the text pays homage to Yī Yǐn's decoctions as an inspiration for doctors and medical authors more than a dozen centuries later is clearly not enough to support a claim that the entire *Fǔxíngjué* is an authentic copy of a text that contains his formulas.

2.8 Other Evidence for the *Tāngyèjīng*

Having exhausted the limits of information to be found among the Máoshān Daoists, let us climb back aboard our Chinese Medicine History Train and chug along until we arrive in the early Táng dynasty. Our next stop is a quick visit with the famous Sūn Sīmiǎo himself in his retirement on "Medicine King Mountain" 藥王山 *Yàowángshān*. The reason for our visit, besides the scenery and the chance to meet Master Sūn's pet dragon and tiger, is a rare mention of Yī Yǐn in the introductory essay to Scroll 26 of Sūn Sīmiǎo's *Qiānjīn yìfāng* 《千金翼方》 ("Appended Formulas Worth a Thousand in Gold," published in 682) on "Selecting [Acupuncture and Moxibustion] Points." A search of received Hàn through Táng dynasty literature has revealed this as the only other reference to Yī Yǐn's decoctions, besides the above-mentioned references in the Hàn bibliographic catalogue and in the *Zhēnjiǔ jiǎyǐjīng* by Huángfǔ Mì from the third century. Here is what Master Sūn has to say:

> 吾十有八而志學於醫，今年過百歲，研綜經方，推究孔穴，所疑更多矣。竊聞尋古人伊尹湯液，依用炎農本草；扁鵲針灸，一准黃帝雷公。
>
> *I have set my mind almost exclusively on studying medicine and am now more than a hundred years old. Having studied and assembled the classical formulas and scrutinized the [acupuncture and moxibustion] holes and points, still my doubts are greater than ever. I have*

heard when tracing back the ancient Yī Yǐn's decoctions that he relied on [Emperor] Yán the Farmer's materia medica, while Biǎn Què's acupuncture and moxibustion was singularly aligned with the Yellow Emperor and Léigōng.

While this passage offers us no new information, it is at least a rare trace, not followed by any other mention of Yī Yǐn in the context of medicinal decoctions until the late twelfth century! This contrasts with a full 7,394 references to him in the literature from the Sòng dynasty alone, but all to his role as a politician in the early years of the Shāng dynasty.[5] Beginning in the twelfth century, a few isolated texts like *Yīshuō* 《醫說》 ("Explanations of Medicine," published in 1189, by Zhāng Gāo 張杲) mention Yī Yǐn's decoctions as a source for classical formula literature in passing, but without contributing any additional information or quoting from an actual text. And even these rare cases are only cursory references that obviously just repeat the original claim by Huángfǔ Mì translated above.

2.9 A Daoist Monk, a French Explorer, and a Doctor Caught in Storms

Given the complete absence of additional evidence in the following centuries, we can fully open the throttle of the History Train and lean back for a long nap, until we arrive all the way at the very beginning of the twentieth century in Dūnhuáng 敦煌, a remote western outpost of the late Qīng empire at the edge of the Gobi desert.

Beginning in the Hàn dynasty but flourishing particularly during the Táng, this frontier garrison had become a sprawling and active

[5] This number is the result of a search for "伊尹" in the Sòng dynasty literature on the digital archive Kanripo, accessed on October 8, 2020, here: https://www.kanripo.org/search?filter=宋&query=伊尹&type=DYNASTY.

religious and commercial hub on the Silk Road, connecting the western outskirts of the Chinese empire to Central Asia. Until its decline after the collapse of the Táng dynasty in the tenth century, it was also the location of an active Buddhist monastic community that created tens of thousands of paintings, murals, statues, and literary works. Having become a popular pilgrimage site, this community created and worked and worshipped in a network of more than a thousand caves now known as the Mògāo Caves 莫高窟 or "caves of the Thousand Buddhas" 千佛洞, of which less than half still exist. The archaeological significance of this site as a whole first received the attention of European explorers in 1879, when an expedition led and financed by Count Béla Széchenyi visited the caves.

In 1900, a local Daoist monk and the self-proclaimed caretaker of the area, Wáng Yuánlù 王圓籙, followed a wisp of cigarette smoke to discover a hidden door in one of the remaining 492 cave temples. Behind this door, which had been sealed for about a thousand years, he discovered a room filled with literally tens of thousands of documents dating from the fifth through tenth centuries that have revolutionized our understanding of all fields of Chinese history, from religion to medicine to politics. To protect this treasure trove during the political chaos of the late Qīng dynasty and a regional peasant rebellion, local officials had the cave resealed in 1904 since they lacked the resources to record, transport, and analyze this important cultural discovery, with the monk put in charge of its preservation.[6]

On March 12, 1907, the British explorer Aurel Stein arrived in Dūnhuáng to investigate the ruined cave temples, only to have the local officials deny that they knew of anything of archaeological value to be found among the ruins. It was only through a foreign

[6] See Jiqing Wang, "Aurel Stein's Dealings with Wang Yuanlu and Chinese Officials in Dunhuang in 1907," in *International Dunhuang Project News* 30, pp. 1–6. (Retrieved from the British Museum National Archives on October 9, 2020).

trader from Urumchi that Stein happened to hear about the recently discovered library cave, which he promptly visited but found locked, with the only key held by the monk Wáng Yuánlù who was away on alms rounds. Finally, on May 23rd, Stein and his Chinese assistant managed to connect with Wáng and gain access to the anteroom of the cave and to a selection of manuscripts that the monk had moved out of the library cave for their inspection. Over the following week, this pile was promptly and secretly carried off to Stein's encampment nearby under cover of night, in exchange for generous payments to Wáng. After a week of this, Wáng reluctantly and in exchange for more silver, granted Stein access to the actual library cave, which convinced Stein that he had to attempt to take possession of the whole lot. Amid political upheaval and in fear of diphtheria and the threat of detection by the authorities, who he had convinced that he was just pursuing a harmless hobby, Stein scrambled to assemble seventeen cases of treasures before hastily leaving the region on June 12th. His assistant subsequently managed to whisk away another 230 bundles with close to 3,000 texts, in a stealthy nighttime operation on camelback. In total, Aurel Stein was able to remove around 7,000 manuscripts and another 6,000 fragments from the library cave, for a nominal amount of silver. These texts eventually ended up in the British Museum where they are housed to this day.

Only months later, the highly skilled French sinologist Paul Pelliot was able to acquire another almost 10,000 other manuscripts, which he had carefully selected by spending several weeks inside the "library cave" at Dūnhuáng itself, doing intense textual research on site with his remarkable classical Chinese language skills. These texts were transported to France and are now housed in Paris. After these two massive lootings of Chinese cultural treasures in the fine tradition of Western colonialism, it was a further two full years before the Chinese imperial government, then in its final years of existence, finally caught wind of this tragic loss, and stopped the bleeding by moving the remaining estimated one fifth of the manuscripts to Běijīng in 1910. Before the national government stepped in, however, the capitalist monk Wáng apparently hid and sold many more manuscripts to local and international customers, including to Japan and Russia, where some manuscripts remain today. How many texts were lost in these years is unknown.

Among this wealth of texts that had been sealed away for roughly a thousand years in the Mògāo library cave, around 83 manuscripts, containing 75 different texts (some are duplicates or parts of a single text), have been found to be medically relevant, covering topics like diagnostics, acupuncture and moxibustion, materia medica, and formula literature. These have been published in modern critical annotated editions in Chinese, most notably Cóng Chūnyǔ 從春雨, ed., *Dūnhuáng zhōngyīyào quánshū* 《敦煌中醫藥全書》 ("Complete Collection of Chinese Medical Manuscripts from Dūnhuáng," published in 1994), the main source text for my own translation. While some of these sources have been discussed in English in a volume edited by Vivienne Lo and Christopher Cullen, published in 2005 and titled *Medieval Chinese Medicine: The Dunhuang Medical Manuscripts*, no complete English translation of this literary treasure exists.

After reading this elaborate story of the Dūnhuáng manuscripts, you are probably asking yourself why we have stopped the History Train here and what this story has to do with the topic of this Preface, namely the history of the *Fǔxíngjué*? Firstly, this text is not included in the numbered lists of manuscripts familiar to any student of Dūnhuáng manuscripts, identified either with an "S" plus number, in the case of manuscripts purchased by Aurel Stein and preserved to this day in the British Museum in London, or with a "P" plus number, for those manuscripts that were collected from Dūnhuáng by Paul Pelliot, currently stored in Paris. So, it is not a text whose contents were ever examined and recorded by either of these two Western explorers. Its existence as part of the Dūnhuáng manuscript collection is also not verified by any outside source and was not known to any researchers until the 1960s.

This is where the Zhāng family of doctors joins our cast of actors. Here is one account by the doctor Zhāng Dàchāng 張大昌, as recorded in the preface to his original publication of the text. It must be pointed out that this story contradicts another account according to which his grandfather purchased the text in 1915 when he visited Dūnhuáng in his official role as stablemaster for the national cavalry:

> *In 1918, my grandfather Zhāng Wònán 張偓南 went to Lánzhōu 蘭州 to see a friend and set aside time specifically to visit the Thousand Buddha Caves in Dūnhuáng. Because of a great windstorm, he spent the night lodging with a Daoist monk, who he struck up a conversation with. When his host found out that my grandfather practiced medicine, he took out a manuscript scroll and said: 'What is written here are all secret techniques and medicinal formulas for practicing medicine and treating illness. I have used these in the past and found them to be extremely effective. This is a text that I have retrieved from one of the Thousand Buddha Caves. If you are interested, take out 50 silver dollars and I can sell it to you.' Fearing a setup, my grandfather initially claimed not to have any money on him and only concluded this transaction right before his departure.*[7]

According to Zhāng Dàchāng as our only source and with no way of verifying this information externally, this is how his grandfather, Zhāng Wònán, came into possession of this text. According to the

[7] See Wáng Xuětái 王雪苔, *Fǔxíngjué zàngfǔ yòngyào fǎyào jiàozhù kǎozhèng* 《辅行诀脏腑用药法要》校注考证 (A textual analysis of *Fǔxíngjué zàngfǔ yòngyào fǎyào*, collated and annotated), Rénmín jūnyī chūbǎnshè 人民军医出版社, 2008, p. 135.

grandson, the elder Zhāng then hid it away as a family treasure for many decades before passing it on to his grandson Zhāng Dàchāng, who studied, memorized, and mastered the contents of the text and in turn passed this information on to a group of disciples. During the Cultural Revolution, Zhāng Dàchāng claims, the original scroll was destroyed in 1966, so that he was forced to reconstruct its contents from memory to create a handwritten copy, which he submitted in 1974 as a "barefoot doctor" to the China Academy of Chinese Medicine in Běijīng. The text then finally received the attention of numerous researchers, most notably the medical historians Wáng Xuětái 王雪苔 and Mǎ Jīxìng 馬繼興, who produced a number of critical editions over the following years and even sent a team of researchers to visit and interview Zhāng Dàchāng and his students. In this context, it is important to note that Zhāng Dàchāng appears to have been the originator of the claim that the *Fǔxíngjué* was not only an authentic medieval formula text but was in fact and in its entirety identical with the long-lost *Tāngyèjīng* as the canonical ancestor of Zhāng Zhòngjǐng's work. We shall return to this claim below.

After detailed evaluation of Zhāng Dàchāng's first handwritten copy and almost two dozen additional versions produced by his students on the basis of their recollections of his teachings, all of which were published in a single volume in 2008,[8] at a minimum, the academic consensus among Chinese historians at this point is that the text can be neither an original work composed by Táo Hóngjǐng, as claimed on its title page, nor that we should simply dismiss it, in spite of the lack of any physical evidence, as a modern forgery based on a single man's account. Instead, the truth, and possible date for

[8] See Zhāng Dàchāng 張大昌 and Qián Chāochén 錢超塵, *Fǔxíngjué wǔzàng yòngyào fǎyào chuánchéngjí* 《辅行诀五臟用药法要》 傳承集 (Collected Transmissions of *Fǔxíngjué wǔzàng yòngyào fǎyào*), Xuéyuàn chūbǎnshè 學苑出版社, 2008. This book includes the complete text of 21 different editions!

its creation, lie somewhere in between. The fact that the *Fǔxíngjué* is included in several critical editions of Dūnhuáng medical manuscripts[9] demonstrates that the leading medical historians in China do treat it as a historically significant text that they believe to have been composed in the medieval period, in the centuries between Táo Hóngjǐng's death in 536 CE and the Northern Sòng dynasty (960–1127 CE). Given the vast amount of research and expertise that these historians have gathered in the decades since its discovery, I humbly suggest that we follow their lead and respect these results.

At the same time, a word of caution is in order since the bar for what is accepted as solid historical evidence tends to be set much higher by Western historians than by their more generous Chinese counterparts. I suspect that this is the real reason why the *Fǔxíngjué* is not a text that has received any attention by Western historians, and it is also the reason why I resisted requests to translate it for many years. In fact, I cannot imagine a Western-trained historian taking a single person's word and their hand-written copy produced from memory, with no outside evidence at all, as irrefutable proof for the existence of a historical text supposedly dating fifteen hundred years back in history, much less reading that text as identical to yet another long lost text that is an additional five hundred years older yet, on the basis of the passages that I have shared with you above. But let us get back on the History Train and continue on our journey.

[9] See, for example, Cóng Chūnyǔ's 從春雨 *Dūnhuáng zhōngyīyào quánshū* 《敦煌中醫藥全書》 ("Complete Collection of Chinese Medical Manuscripts from Dūnhuáng," published in 1994); Mǎ Jīxìng's 馬繼興 *Dūnhuáng gǔyījí kǎoshì* 敦煌古醫籍考釋 ("Philological Study of the Ancient Dūnhuáng Medical Records," published in 1988); and Mǎ Jīxìng et als, *Dūnhuáng yīyào wénxiàn jíjiào* 敦煌醫藥文獻輯校 ("Collected Collations of the Medical Texts from Dūnhuáng," published in 1998).

2.10 A Creative Medical Fiction Writer in 1940s Hongkong

Before crossing the Big Pond to arrive in my studio in the Pacific Northwest rain forest, we have to put our History Train in reverse and make a quick detour to Hong Kong in the 1940s. Muddying the waters of textual history to cause yet more confusion is another book with the title *Tāngyèjīng* 湯液經 (Classic of Decoctions), which was first published in Hong Kong by Yáng Shìyǐn 楊師尹 in 1948 and reprinted twice. This book self-confidently claims to be a reconstruction of Yī Yǐn's original "Classic of Decoctions" as the ancestor of Zhāng Zhòngjǐng's work. Given the spurious historical evidence that the text is based on, however, it is only fair to say that it was "created" by Yáng on the basis of Zhāng Zhòngjǐng's writings, Wáng Shūhé's 王叔和 *Màijīng* 脈經 (Pulse Classic, late third century CE) and Sūn Sīmiǎo's 孫思邈 *Qiānjīn yìfāng* 千金翼方 (Appended Formulas Worth a Thousand in Gold, 682 CE). Because it extrapolates textual connections that are historically unverifiable, it is safe to simply dismiss this additional text as a modern creation of no historical value.

3

Significance in Contemporary China and Global Transmission

Now we are finally getting ready to cross various oceans and deserts to arrive at our final destinations, the contemporary US, Europe, and Australia. In the last decade or so, a small number of international practitioners of Chinese medicine have begun to teach the contents of the *Fǔxíngjué* around the world. Noteworthy is Abel Gläser's *Fǔ Xíng Jué: Procédés subtils des Mouvements de l'Étoile Alcor* (Institut Liang Shen, 2019), a translation of the text in French that is unfortunately not widely known. This recent publication includes the Chinese text of the *Fǔxíngjué* in simplified characters, a solid literal translation, and insightful commentary. To clinical practitioners who can read French, this book can serve as an important source of information on the text. It contains a host of charts, a more clinical orientation than the present book, and a lengthy discussion on astronomy, based on the author's reading of the character 輔 *fǔ* not as "helpful" but as the Chinese name of a star called Alcor in the handle of the Big Dipper. As such, it is an important resource for practitioners unable to read Chinese.

Other than this book and the already-mentioned academic article by Wang Shumin that I will briefly review below, the only access to the *Fǔxíngjué* in Western languages has been through private seminars. Perhaps influenced by Zhāng Dàchāng's claims, the contents of the *Fǔxíngjué* have become known in some Western circles as identical with an ancient "*Tāngyèjīng*" that is claimed to have been the ancestor of Zhāng Zhòngjǐng's work. In sharp contrast, it is important to note here that the major teachers of the *jīngfāng* style of medicine in China, like Huáng Huáng 黃煌, Fù Yánlíng 傅延齡, and Féng Shìlún

馮世綸, do not include the *Fŭxíngjué* or any "*Tāngyèjīng* system" or "Tāngyèjīng formulas" as a central element in their teaching, much less emphasize this text as essential to an understanding of *jīngfāng* medicine and foundational in their analysis of Zhāng Zhòngjǐng's formulas.[10]

The clearest evidence for this approach to the *Fŭxíngjué* in China is an actual book by Féng Shìlún titled *Zhōngguó tāngyè jīngfāng: Shānghán zábìnglùn chuánzhēn* 《中國湯液經方：傷寒雜病論傳真》 ("Classical Formulas for Decoctions from China: The True Transmission of the *Treatise on Cold Damage and Miscellaneous Diseases*"), which was published in 2005. Contrary to what you may think after reading this title, this book is not about the *Tāngyèjīng* at all and only mentions the *Fŭxíngjué* in passing. It discusses the *Tāngyèjīng* as an actual classical text in a mere page and a half of a total of 558 pages and never equates it with the *Fŭxíngjué*. The main thrust of the brief passage on the *Tāngyè jīngfǎ* is two-fold: First, a collection of formulas called *Tāngyè jīngfǎ* may have been one of the sources used by Zhāng Zhòngjǐng, along with the *Shénnóng běncǎo jīng* and many other now lost formula texts that he gathered together and studied to create his own work. Second, traces of this lost text appear in the *Fŭxíngjué*, especially in the section on the Six Spirit and Two Major and Minor "Dawning" formulas, which are strikingly similar to Zhāng Zhòngjǐng's writings. As such, Féng Shìlún quotes Mǎ Jìxìng in stating that "the formulas in that section of [the *Fŭxíngjué*] are similar to [Zhāng] Zhòngjǐng's work, and this can serve as evidence that these two are both derived from a *Tāngyè jīngfǎ*."[11] Nowhere,

---

[10] This information is based on personal communication with three leading Western voices on jīngfāng medicine who have studied extensively with these teachers in China and observed and practiced under their direct clinical supervision: Sharon Weizenbaum, Michael Max, and Eran Even.

[11] Féng Shìlún 馮世綸, *Zhōngguó tāngyè jīngfāng: Shānghán zábìnglùn chuánzhēn* 《中國湯液經方：傷寒雜病論傳真》 ("Classical Formulas for Decoctions from

however, does this book equate the content of the *Fŭxíngjué* as a whole with this mysterious lost "classical methods of decoctions." It is also significant that the other content of the *Fŭxíngjué*, such as the remaining formulas and the chart and list that associate the twenty-five medicinal substances with the five flavors and *wŭxíng*, is not mentioned at all.

The purpose of the present introduction is not at all to question or deny the clinical value of the formulas and of the innovative classificatory system of medicinal substances in the *Fŭxíngjué*. Many students of Chinese medicine have found the way in which this text combines the theory of *wŭxíng* resonances with the clinically oriented formula literature meaningful. As such, this text has provided an approachable entryway to the clinical practice of traditional Chinese medicinal therapy for some practitioners eager to expand their therapeutic repertoire beyond acupuncture and moxibustion and desiring to understand medicinal formulas on a deeper level. This clinical significance is certainly a good reason why this text has received considerable attention from medical historians in China, as a medieval source, since its discovery in the 1970s. It is also the reason why I have decided to take on this translation project, in constant consultation and close collaboration with the experienced *jīngfāng* practitioner Sharon Weizenbaum. It is our sincere hope that readers will find the *Fŭxíngjué* formulas and medicinal classification scheme useful as one more tool to employ in their clinical practice and as a stepping-stone on their journey towards becoming an ever more proficient Chinese medicine doctor in the proud tradition of the Chinese scholar-physicians.

Before concluding this section, however, we must return to the academic article already mentioned above by the Chinese medical

---

China: The True Transmission of the *Treatise on Cold Damage and Miscellaneous Diseases*"), p. 5–6.

historian Wáng Shūmín 王淑民.[12] Until now, this was the only English publication on this subject, albeit a translation of a Chinese article. While that article follows academic consensus and dates the *Fǔxíngjué* to after Táo Hóngjǐng's death, it focuses on discussing some of the formulas contained in the text as representative of what she calls as "Tangyejing/Fuxingjue tradition," which Wáng clearly sees as predating and informing Zhāng Zhòngjǐng's writings. She states the following about the *Fǔxíngjué*:

> *According to modern research, however, it is verified as a work compiled by Tao's disciples according to his doctrines, which might have been completed some time during the period from Tao's death to the Sui and Tang dynasties (ca. 540–800). Through detailed research I have found that the medical formulae recorded in this manuscript are mainly records from Tangye jingfa, and that the structure of its compilation has provided the first thread for modern research into Tangye's lost texts.*[13]

Unfortunately, Wáng Shūmín's article is not a comprehensive introduction to the text and therefore does not discuss its long and problematic history or fully address the question of a hypothetical "Tāngyèjīng tradition" as preceding Zhāng Zhòngjǐng's work. It is important to keep in mind that the publication in which this article appears is aimed at an advanced academic audience presumed to be familiar with existing Chinese publications on Dūnhuáng manuscripts. And when read in the context of all existing research on the *Fǔxíngjué*, Dr. Wáng makes a valuable contribution by analyzing the content of the text from a clinical perspective and by juxtaposing

---

[12] See her article, "*Tangy jingfa* (Canonical Methods for Brews and Decoctions) 湯液經法: A Lost Text Recorded in the *Hanshu* Bibliography," in Vivienne Lo and Christopher Cullen, eds, *Medieval Chinese Medicine: The Dunhuang Medical Manuscripts* (Routledge, 2005), pp. 322–344.

[13] Ibid., p. 324

it to Zhāng Zhòngjǐng's work. She is the first and only medical historian, in China or the West, however, to associate this text in any way with a lost textual tradition around the *Tāngyè jīngfǎ* ("classical methods of decoctions"). As such, when this article is taken as one's only source of information on the *Fǔxíngjué*, and without also taking into consideration the standard reading of the text, it can unfortunately leave the less informed reader with a false impression about the relationship between this text and the *Tāngyèjīng*.

For a more accurate and historically oriented evaluation of the *Fǔxíngjué*, it is essential that we supplement her article with, and read it in the context of, the much more thorough and comprehensive treatment that the *Fǔxíngjué* has received in numerous Chinese academic publications, many under the aegis of her mentor Mǎ Jīxìng 馬繼興. One of the main publications on the Dūnhuáng medical manuscripts is a compilation on which Dr. Wáng is actually listed as co-editor: Mǎ Jīxìng et als, *Dūnhuáng yīyào wénxiàn jíjiào* 敦煌醫藥文獻輯校 ("Collected Collations of the Medical Texts from Dūnhuáng"), published in 1998.[14] In that collection, the *Fǔxíngjué* is repeatedly described in both the introduction to the text and then in Mǎ Jīxìng's detailed analysis and discussion of dating the text that follows the transcription, as a Dūnhuáng manuscript that must date from the period between Táo Hóngjǐng's death and the beginning of the Northern Sòng dynasty (960 CE). Nowhere in the introduction or the lengthy discussion is the text identified with a lost *Tāngyèjīng*! In fact, the *Tāngyèjīng* is only mentioned once in the entire chapter on the *Fǔxíngjué* in this collection of Dūnhuáng manuscripts, namely as one of the ancient texts cited in the text itself. While Mǎ Jīxìng does recognize and analyze the classical nature of the medicinal substances used, and the parallelism to some of Zhāng Zhòngjǐng's formulas, this does not lead him to conclude that we are dealing

[14] See pp. 169–206 in that book.

with a Hàn period text or even a text that cites a Hàn dynasty source. Far from this, he argues eloquently and conclusively that the references to Hàn and post-Hàn doctors, the terminology of disease names and medicinals, as well as certain character variations that were only common during the Táng and Sòng periods, make it clear that the text is not a modern forgery but fits perfectly into the style and content of Dūnhuáng medical manuscripts and must therefore be understood as a medieval text, dating to the sixth century at the earliest.

Similarly, the collection of Dūnhuáng medical manuscripts in a critical edition by Cóng Chūnyǔ 從春雨 titled *Dūnhuáng zhōngyīyào quánshū* 《敦煌中醫藥全書》 ("Complete Collection of Chinese Medical Manuscripts from Dūnhuáng"), published in 1994, also does not mention any connection between this text and a possible lost *Tāngyèjīng* tradition as ancestral to Zhāng Zhòngjǐng's work. As a matter of fact, this book even quotes Wáng Shūmín herself as concluding:

> *It is not a work created by Táo Hóngjǐng himself but was created by later writers who collated his teachings.*

At the danger of repeating myself, I am providing this information here not to question the value of this manuscript as a whole or to question the applicability of its formulas in the contemporary clinical practice of Chinese medicine. If the formulas work and the model of explaining and conceptualizing the relationship between medicinal substances and formulas, on the one hand, and the theory of resonances of five dynamic agents, flavors, and *zàng* organs, on the other hand, are meaningful, by all means it should be taught and transmitted. And that is why I have created the present book. My desire is merely to provide the necessary details here for the problems around the date and history of transmission of this text, which have resulted in a large number of different versions with considerable discrepancies and omissions or additions. Ultimately, these academic discussions may well be irrelevant to practitioners who are just looking to expand their toolbox through the addition of the forty-three formulas listed in this sweet little text and its theoretical model for conceptualizing medicinals.

The following sections provide a bit more textual evidence for dating the text, as well as a brief survey of the major differences between the various manuscripts. Readers who are more interested in just the clinical applications of this text are invited to skip the following pages and dive right into the translation of the text itself.

4

Dating the *Fǔxíngjué* on Account of Language and Content

There are a number of terms, concepts, and expressions found throughout the different textual layers of the *Fǔxíngjué* that clearly show that this text could not have been written and compiled until many centuries after the fall of the Hàn dynasty and Zhāng Zhòngjǐng's lifetime, and even after Táo Hóngjǐng's passing. Given the classical style of the formulas, the substances used, and the textual parallels to Zhāng Zhòngjǐng's work in some layers of the text, it is indeed possible or even likely that some of the formulas found in the text are older and are derived from or share a common ancestor with Zhāng Zhòngjǐng's source or sources. Nevertheless, such an incorporation of older material is typical of every historical medical text in China, since it has always been part of the scholarly and medical tradition to rely on earlier knowledge instead of rejecting it wholesale and creating something drastically new, as is more common in the history of Western science and medicine. The mere fact that a few formulas or certain sections of the *Fǔxíngjué* have strong textual parallels with a Hàn dynasty text cannot by any stretch of the imagination prove that the text as a whole is that old, or even less that it actually predates the other text. To determine the date of a text as a whole, we must determine the date of its newest layers, not its oldest.

4.1 Texts, Titles, and Doctors Mentioned and Cited in the Text

Before diving into the details of the language of the text, let us start with the easiest piece of information for dating the *Fǔxíngjué*, namely the texts, titles, and doctors it mentions and quotes. The text clearly cites several chapters from the *Nèijīng* literally, both *Sùwèn* and *Língshū*, sometimes identifying them as "The Classic states" 經云, but other times just incorporating them into the text. This is fairly convincing evidence that the text as a whole cannot be taken as an intermediate step between the *Néijīng* and Zhāng Zhòngjǐng's work since the original layers of *Sùwèn* and *Língshū* were taking shape in their current form only in the second half of the Hàn dynasty. More importantly, the *Fǔxíngjué* also mentions the *Shānghánlùn* by name, as well as many famous doctors from the Hàn and post-Hàn period, even including the above-cited Huángfǔ Mì. So how could this text be identical with the *Tāngyèjīng* when it mentions Huángfǔ Mì, who names that ancient title in a single obscure reference? Regarding the supposed comments by Táo Hóngjǐng, I will repeat, the mere fact that the text claims to have been compiled by Táo or that some of the comments are credited to him does not mean that he was the originator of either the comments or the text as a whole. The following discussion will show why we must date the *Fǔxíngjué* to the centuries after his death.

4.2 Taboo Characters and Other Dated Terms

One of the most important tools employed by Chinese archaeologists and scholars for dating texts, or individual layers within a text, is to identify the presence of taboo characters or note their avoidance, in Chinese 避諱 *bì huì* ("avoiding a taboo"). These are specific characters (and their etymological derivatives) that ordinary mortals were not allowed to use in any given era because they were part of the emperor's name. As such, the intentional avoidance of a character and the replacement with a commonly used substitute strongly suggests that a passage was either composed or copied during the particular era when that character was taboo. On the flipside, the presence of a taboo character indicates that the text was not compiled or copied during that era and most likely predates that taboo, since these changes in nomenclature often came to be permanent. Of course, it is always possible that an educated scribe who was aware of these taboos intentionally observed or violated them, or *corrected* or *restored* a text back to its original version in the creation of a forgery, to make it appear like a more valuable and authentic antique. Nevertheless, investigating the presence or absence of taboo characters is one of the main tools employed by Chinese historians in their attempt to date manuscripts like those from Dūnhuáng.

The most notable example of this character taboo in the *Fǔxíngjué* is probably the fact that the text has kept the traditional name Xuán Wǔ 玄武 (Dark Warrior) in the formula for Xuán Wǔ Tāng 玄武湯 (Dark Warrior Decoction) instead of replacing it with what most practitioners have come to know as Zhēn Wǔ Tāng 真武湯 (True Warrior Decoction). Since the character 玄 *xuán* became a taboo character in the year 1012 by imperial declaration due to its association with the name of an ancestor of the Sòng imperial lineage, its presence in the *Fǔxíngjué* strongly suggests that the text was compiled and copied prior to this date. Now this may confuse you since we are so programmed to think of the *Shānghánlùn* as a Hàn dynasty text, and in that text the formula name is written as Zhēn Wǔ Tāng. Thus, you are probably wondering why that text would observe a character taboo from the Sòng period when the *Fǔxíngjué*, which is presumably many centuries later, would not! The reason for this is that the received standard versions of the *Shānghánlùn* that most scholars and practitioners today work with are all based on editions that postdate the edits and "corrections" during the Sòng period. This is just one example to demonstrate the historical significance of archaeologically discovered manuscripts like the Dūnhuáng texts, which predate the changes that the received literature underwent during the Sòng and later periods.

Let us look at one more example of a term that can help us with the dating of the *Fǔxíngjué*: the medicinal that the text refers to as 署蕷 *shǔyù*. This substance is identical with what is known to most TCM practitioners as 山藥 *shānyào* (potato yam, the rhizome of Dioscorea opposita). In texts that predate the mid-Táng period, this substance is consistently referred to as 署蕷 *shǔyù*, but its name was changed in response to a taboo concerning the character 預 *yù* (closely related to the second character of the medicinal's name 蕷 *yù*), part of the personal name of Táng emperor Dàizōng 代宗 (726–779 CE). As a result, the substance became known in the mid-Táng period as 署菜 *shǔcài*, but changed names yet again in response to another taboo against the use of 曙 *shǔ* (related to the first character 署 *shǔ*) in the personal name of Sòng emperor Yīngzōng 英宗 (1032–1067), to the name that we still use today: 山藥 *shānyào*. Thus, we can date formula and materia medica texts, or at least the edition or textual layer in question, by the name which the text uses to refer to this substance. In the case of the *Fǔxíngjué*, the use of the name *shǔyù* in several formulas suggests that these layers of the text predate the mid-eighth century. Specifically, the term is found in only two contexts: First, it occurs twice as a potential substitute for dàzǎo in the Minor and Major Liver-Supplementing Decoctions in the first major section of the text, on the Minor and Major *Zàng*-Supplementing and -Draining Formulas. Second, it is mentioned in the fourth section of the *Fǔxíngjué* in the list of twenty-five medicinals categorized in association with the *wǔxíng*, where shǔyù is listed as the water medicinal of the sour flavor that belongs to metal.

In addition to these taboo characters, there are other particularities in the language of the text that support accepting the *Fǔxíngjué* as an authentic medieval text from among the Dūnhuáng manuscripts. First off, the text preserves some old names for ingredients that are common in early and medieval literature but only rarely found in later texts or in transmitted versions of earlier texts that were edited during the Sòng period. According to Mǎ Jìxìng, different chapters of the *Fǔxíngjué* use a variety of older terms to refer to the ingredient vinegar, rather than employing the later term 醋 *cù*.[15] I disagree with his statement that these various terms (specifically 白截漿 *báizàijiāng* and 苦酒 *kǔjiǔ*) can be directly equated with the modern 醋 *cù* ("vinegar"), and instead translate them more specifically as "fermented rice drink" and "soured rice wine," respectively, or in other words, as varieties of fermented rice drink in different stages of fermentation. My reason is that medieval authors like Gě Hóng 葛洪, Sūn Sīmiǎo 孫思邈, and Wáng Táo 王濤 (author of the *Wàitái mìyào* 外台秘要 "Essential Secrets from the Outer Terrace"), who use both of these terms, also use the character 醋 *cù* and so must be distinguishing in some way between these three substances. But regardless of the particular meaning of each term and the minor differences between them, the fact that the *Fǔxíngjué* does use these terms is yet another argument that supports a medieval date for at least those layers of the text that contain them. Taken

[15] See his concluding remarks in Mǎ Jìxìng et als, *Dūnhuáng yīyào wénxiàn jíjiào* 敦煌醫藥文獻輯校, pp. 196–7.

together, these two phrases appear in Sections One on "Differentiating Patterns of *Zàng* Organ Disease," Three on the "Five Formulas for Supplementing the Five *Zàng* Organs" and Five on the "Classical Treatments for External Contraction." To conclude this discussion on terminology, the language used in the *Fǔxíngjué* is one of the key arguments that support a medieval date for this text, rather than interpreting it as a forgery from the twentieth century.

4.3 Dating the *Fǔxíngjué* by Medical Content: The Meaning of "Classical"

Beyond the particularities of the language employed in the text, there are other findings that we can use to try and narrow the date of this text, suggesting limits both for its earliest possible composition and for the latest date of compilation.

First and probably most obvious to practitioners trained in the "classical" or "canonical" tradition of Chinese medicine, the medicinal substances called for in the formulas in this book will all be familiar to Zhāng Zhòngjǐng fans or readers of the *Divine Farmer's Classic of Materia Medica*. Moreover, they also accord with medicinal ingredients that we see mentioned in archaeologically discovered manuscripts from the Hàn dynasty. Looked at from another angle, the difference is striking between the medicinals employed here and the much larger range of substances used in standard texts from the Táng dynasty and later, a development that is related to the extensive contact that occurred between China and Central Asia and areas further west along the Silk Road during that time. This fact suggests that, in spite of its supposed discovery in the far Western reaches of the Chinese empire in Dūnhuáng, the *Fǔxíngjué* was not a text that had been compiled locally in this multicultural desert oasis but actually had originated elsewhere in China before being transported to and sealed away in the Library Cave of Dūnhuáng for around a thousand years.

Nevertheless, the exclusive use of "classical" medicinals in the formulas should not cause us to claim a classical age for the text itself. Quite to the contrary, the fact that the text repeatedly and self-consciously includes phrases like 經方 *jīngfāng* "classical formulas," 經法 *jīngfǎ* "classical methods," and even 舊經 *jiùjīng* "old classics," is actually an argument for a more recent date. Zhāng Zhòngjǐng himself certainly did not proclaim himself to be the creator or transmitter of a "classic" or "classical methods" or "classical formulas." Thus, these terms are not found in any of the early texts, with one exception in Zhāng Zhòngjǐng's preface where he laments: "When I look at today's doctors, they do not study and ponder the meaning of the Classics in order to advance what they know." Writing at the end of the Hàn dynasty, Zhāng Zhòngjǐng was already aware of the elevated status of the "Inner Classic" (*Nèijīng* 內經), "Classic of Difficulties" (*Nànjīng* 難經), and "Divine Farmer's Classic of Materia Medica" (*Shénnóng běncǎo jīng* 神農本草經) and was referring to this body of literature. Nevertheless, it would have never occurred to him to call his own style of formulas a "classical method." In contrast, references to "classical formulas" or a "classical method" begin to be commonplace in the writings of medieval scholars like Sūn Sīmiǎo, where the authors use them to distinguish an older tradition of medical practice from the numerous innovations of the times, many of which were related to the influx of medical information from Central Asia and beyond, riding on the coattails of Buddhism. Given the frequent references to "classical formulas" and "classical methods" in the *Fǔxíngjué*, as well as the exclusive use of Hàn-dynasty ingredients in the formulas, I suggest that we interpret the use of the character *jīng* 經 in these compound terms as referring not to some ancient Classic of Decoctions from the Shāng or even Hàn dynasty but to what seemed "classical" to the medieval creators of the text, namely old-style formulas that stood out due to their exclusive use of traditional Hàn-dynasty medicinal ingredients.

Let us now look more closely at the theoretical concepts that we can detect in the *Fǔxíngjué*, to see whether the meaning of "classical" in these so-called "classical formulas" went beyond just the choice of materia medica they employed. The following discussion will not only contribute to our understanding of the meaning of "classical" in the text, but is also important for our attempts to date the text.

While clinical practitioners may be better equipped to evaluate the "classical" nature of the formulas in the *Fǔxíngjué* intuitively, as a medical historian specializing in Hàn to Sòng medical literature I bring a different skillset to the table that gives me different insights. To begin with, I am keenly aware from my decades of translating and researching Táng to Sòng formula literature, years of researching a PhD dissertation, and writing a number of specialized books in the field, that all the received formula texts from this period are compilations instead of the creative work of a single author. During this period, the so-called "authors" who compiled and composed these texts, culminating in a specific date of publication, were certainly not themselves the creators of these formulas who had developed innovative treatments on the basis of their personal clinical experience. Instead, they were compilers and collectors, members of the literate elite who had access to medical texts, still hand-copied or perhaps even memorized and orally transmitted at this time. As they often express in prefaces or statements in the text, these men were motivated by the tremendous loss of medical knowledge that had occurred in the centuries of warfare and destruction between the collapse of the Hàn dynasty and the reunification of China under the short-lived Suí dynasty, i.e., in the years 220 to 581 CE. Even though traditional Chinese authors rarely credit their sources in the way modern academics are trained to do, the more one becomes familiar with the key texts, or learns to employ digital search tools, the more one realizes that these texts are but compilations of layer upon layer of older material. This fact has become abundantly clear to me in my most recent work with Qí Zhòngfǔ's 齊仲甫 *Nǚkē bǎiwèn* 女科百問 ("Hundred Questions on Gynecology," published in 1220 CE). In this text, practically every theoretical statement and formula is either a direct quote or a slightly altered or updated version of an earlier textual layer, in the vast majority of cases without crediting the source. Similarly, even without doing this painstaking detective work, it would be negligent, if not misleading, if we were to present Sūn Sīmiǎo as the author and sole creator of all the formulas in his famous *Bèijí qiānjīn yàofāng* 備急千金要方 ("Essential Formulas Worth a Thousand in Gold to Prepare for Emergencies). While we may refer to "Sūn Sīmiǎo's formulas" or "Táo Hóngjǐng's clinical advice" in the heat of teaching or out of convenience, we should always keep in mind that the authors of classical and medieval medical texts in general, and of formularies in particular, were rarely medical practitioners in our modern sense of medical professionals in full-time clinical practice, like the "scholar-physicians" (儒醫 *rúyī*) who began to emerge during the Sòng dynasty. Quite to the contrary, the professionals who practiced medicine as a family tradition were much more likely to keep access to their treatments tightly controlled and only pass their knowledge on to a small circle of family members or disciples, in the interest of protecting their clan's livelihood. Nevertheless, even though a considerable percentage of the content of these traditional texts was probably much older than the date of publication of the whole, we must read these texts as products of that date since their compilers chose to extract and combine passages from previous works in such a manner as to support and promote their contemporaneous understanding of medical knowledge. Thus, for example, we cannot read the *Huángdì nèijīng* or the *Shénnóng běncǎo jīng* as Warring States texts, even though they clearly contain older layers that precede the founding of the Hàn dynasty. When read as a whole, these two classics reflect an understanding of medicine that is clearly more advanced than archaeological discoveries like the Mǎwángduī medical manuscripts from 168 BCE. This is precisely why the discovery of manuscripts has revolutionized our understanding of medical history: As a result of these precisely dated archaeological findings, we have, through comparison, had to drastically adjust the dating of received and transmitted texts that have traditionally claimed to be far older than we now know them to be. As a medical historian, this question of the creation and evolution of medical knowledge is something that is always present in the back of my mind.

4.4 The Invention of Pharmacology?

With this caveat in place, what immediately struck me about the *Fǔxíngjué* as truly innovative, and therefore as a significant contribution to the early history of Chinese medicine, was the creative synthesis that takes place in this text between two traditionally separate genres of Chinese medical literature: Formulary literature on the one hand, and the theoretical classics on the other. Zhāng Zhòngjǐng obviously utilized a theoretical concept in his writings, albeit without ever spelling it out for us, namely what are known in Chinese as the 六經 *liùjīng* and translated in English as "Six Conformations," "Six Syndromes," "Six Levels," "Six Warps," or my personal favorite, Sharon Weizenbaum's "Six Thing-a-ma-jigs."[16] As

[16] The translation of the term 六經 has caused far too much conflict in contemporary circles of Chinese medicine practitioners. Rather than emphasizing how wrong the other person's "translation" is, wouldn't it be nice if we could all agree that there simply is no single English term that works in this context, and that we should therefore simply start using the Chinese *liùjīng*, as we have learned to do with the word Qì? See Sharon Weizenbaum's illuminating three blog posts for a good recent discussion of this controversy at https://whitepinehealingarts.org/what-does-經-mean/.

Weizenbaum masterfully points out in her commentary to Section Five of the present book, the *liùjīng* as a model for framing the progression of vital Yáng energy through the body, the day, the year, and innumerable other microcosms allows us to make sense of Zhāng Zhòngjǐng's treatments from a deeper theoretically-rooted perspective that can vastly improve clinical outcomes. While Weizenbaum focuses these particular comments on what may be the earliest layer of formulas in the *Fǔxíngjué*, namely the fifth section of the text on the "Classical Treatments for External Contractions of Celestial Movements," which operates within this framework of the *liùjīng*, the *Fǔxíngjué* as a whole stands out to me for its incorporation of the framework of the 五行 *wǔxíng* ("five movements," also translated as "Five Elements," "Five Phases," or "Five Dynamic Agents") and of the five *zàng* organs in resonance with them. The incorporation of this concept of *wǔxíng* resonance between the forces of the macrocosm and the internal proceedings of the microcosm of the body, and the classification of twenty-five medicinal substances within this framework in particular, are what make this text truly unique and path-breaking. It is standard knowledge among medical historians that there is no trace to be found in any of the received texts until the Sòng dynasty for this new way of categorizing materia medica, or of relating the theory of the five *zàng* organs and five "dynamic agents/elements" to formula literature. We may disagree with some of Paul U. Unschuld's views on "systematic" versus "magical" correspondence. However, what he states here in regards to a much later materia medica text, namely the *Běncǎo yǎnyì* 本草衍義 ("Expanded Meaning of the Materia Medica"), a text by Kòu Zōngshì 寇宗奭 from 1116, is extremely relevant to our story:

> *The* pen-ts'ao yen-i *can be seen as a forerunner to the drug works of the Chin-Yüen epoch: Certain elements already indicate the combination of the classical medical theory of the* Huang-ti nei-ching, *that is, the yinyang and Five Phases paradigms of systematic*

> *correspondence—with the practice of actual drug usage. Such a tendency stood in contrast to the preceding contents of pen-ts'ao works in the main tradition; these works were oriented totally for pragmatic use, without any explicit theoretical trimmings. The knowledge expressed in them rested on purely primary experiences or observations and on simple speculations based on the paradigm of magic correspondence.*[17]

In other words, originally *běncǎo* was a completely separate literary genre that was not authored with medical application and clinical relevance in mind.[18] Under the influence of Táo Hóngjǐng's writings, from the sixth century on, *běncǎo* texts incorporated increasing amounts of medical information and were authored and revised and annotated by medical authors, but with purely practical information. According to Unschuld, it was only in the 12th century that materia medica texts even BEGAN to consider how the theory of *wǔxíng* resonance could inform the application of medicinal substances to treat illness in the human body. While Unschuld may eventually be proven to have been off by a century or two, his main point still offers an important correction to those contemporary clinicians who want to read the entire *Fǔxíngjué* as a copy of a lost text from the Hàn dynasty! Without any additional unequivocal supporting evidence, such a view stands in stark contrast to our understanding of the development of Chinese medical history.

Most notably, we look in vain for traces of this new synthesis between materia medica literature and the theory of resonances in any of the other medically oriented texts composed by Táo Hóngjǐng, including his famous revision of the *Shénnóng běncǎojīng*. It is simply inconceivable to me that a highly educated famous person like Táo,

---

[17] See Paul U. Unschuld, *Medicine in China: A History of Pharmaceutics*, p. 81.

[18] See the Introduction to my translation of the *Shénnóng běncǎojīng*, published as "Divine Farmer's Classic of Materia Medica" in 2017.

the revered founder of a religious community and author of a plethora of medical, religious, and alchemical texts that are known to us by title if not by content, had access to this new way of categorizing materia medica and conceptualizing formula architecture and would have only written about it in one text but not shared it in his other writings. This, to me, is the strongest argument for dating the *Fǔxíngjué* in the roughly five centuries after Táo's death.

In addition, one of Táo Hóngjǐng's great contributions in his revision of the *Shénnóng běncǎojīng* was arguably a concern with subtly changing *běncǎo* literature into a literary genre that was clinically useful for practicing physicians or readers consulting it for medical information. I am not even sure it is fair to translate the Chinese term 本草 *běncǎo* (literally "roots and grasses") as "materia medica" prior to Táo Hóngjǐng's involvement in the genre! While the importance of *běncǎo* literature for clinical practice may seem obvious to a modern reader with a standard education in Chinese medicinal substances from a text like *Chinese Herbal Medicine: Materia Medica*,[19] picture yourself as a healer in early China looking for medically relevant information on the substances you were using. Prior to Táo's revision of the *Divine Farmer's Classic of Materia Medica*, how directly useful and applicable would this text have been in its original state? We are so used to approaching this text through the lens of Táo's additions and structural changes that this may even be a difficult question for you to answer. As a matter of fact, it was one of the key motivations for my own translation of the original text that so many contemporary readers are simply unaware of Táo's involvement and the changes he introduced. To briefly review, most importantly, he changed the organization of the entire text, and of the substances discussed in the text: Rather than organizing the text in three volumes on the basis of the traditional upper, middle, and lower

[19] Dan Bensky, Steven Clavey, Erich Stoger, and Andrew Gamble, *Chinese Herbal Medicine: Materia Medica* (Eastland Press, 1990 and 2004).

grades of medicinals, his three volumes consist of an introductory volume containing a lengthy preface by Táo on the "origin of the nature of medicinals," an index of medicinals categorized under eighty-three illnesses and symptoms, and a number of prohibitions; a middle volume where substances are arranged in separate chapters on stones and minerals and on substances derived from herbs and trees, with each subcategorized according to the three grades of the original text; and a third volume on insects, fish, and other animals, fruits and vegetables, and grains and food substances, also subcategorized according to the three grades. Obviously, this makes it much easier for the reader to consult the text and find practical information on a particular substance. In addition, he added extensive clinical information in the actual text, both in his own commentaries and in the "Separate Records by Renowned Physicians" (名醫別錄 *míngyī biélù*). In retrospect, it may be difficult to see how innovative this integration of clinical information into *běncǎo* literature was in Táo's time. For our efforts at contextualizing and dating the *Fǔxíngjué*, however, it is essential that we keep this drastic innovation, which we can date precisely to around 500 CE, in mind. We simply do not have any historical evidence prior to Táo's work of anybody else even thinking about combining *běncǎo* information with formula literature. And we can see from the ubiquitous presence of sections on materia medica in all the major formula collections and of clinical information and medical comments in materia medica literature after this time that this integration of clinical information into *běncǎo* literature by Táo was a hugely influential change that profoundly affected the development of both of these textual genres forever after. In my mind, what makes this historical progression important for our efforts at dating the *Fǔxíngjué* is that the text does in fact combine these two genres, with a central section on individual medicinal substances sandwiched in between different and unrelated sets of formula literature. While especially the section on the Two Dawning and Six Major and Minor Spirit

Formulas is quite possibly based on an earlier source text, it seems highly unlikely that the text as a whole, which in this particular combination is extremely unusual for a work predating Táo's innovative work, could have been composed at an earlier date.

For another perspective, we know from a number of texts in the Daoist religious literature that this way of thinking about treatment as "draining and supplementing the five *zàng* and six *fǔ* organs" became very popular between the Táng and the Sòng period, including even graphic representations of the animal spirits associated with the organs.[20] It was an expression of the emerging "Daoist medicine" that was the result of practitioners combining the clinical application of *zàngfǔ* theory with the authors' religious cultivation as Daoist practitioners. As Zhāng Qíchéng points out in a study of three such texts, there are two insights we can gain from these supposedly later texts, as the result of differences between these texts in comparison to the information of the Six Spirits in the *Fǔxíngjué*: First, after depicting the lung as a white tiger or "tiger-like beast," the heart as the "vermilion bird," and the liver as the dragon, these three texts all depict the spirit animal of the spleen as a phoenix and the kidney as a two-headed white deer. The author suggests that there are two reasons for this association of the kidney with the deer in Daoist literature: First, the kidney is associated with softness and pliability, which is also associated with the inherent nature of the deer in traditional China. Second, and perhaps more importantly, the deer is associated with longevity, and the kidney is the root of earlier heaven. The double head of the deer may be related to the dual nature of the kidneys. A second interesting insight is that the

[20] See Zhāng Qíchéng 張其成, *Wǔzàng liùfǔ bǔxiètú jiěshuō* 五臟六腑補瀉圖解說 ("Explaining the illustrations for supplementing and draining of the five *zàng* and six *fǔ* organs"), in Wáng Shūmín 王淑民 and Vivienne Lo, *Xíngxiàng zhōngyī* 《形象中醫》 ("Visualizing Chinese Medicine") (Renmin weisheng 人民衛生, 2007, 175–181).

sixth spirit in these three Daoist texts is always the turtle-serpent (龜蛇 *guīshé*), in the Daoist texts associated with the gallbladder as the sixth organ and an alternate name for the "Dark Warrior" (玄武 *xuánwǔ*). This is of course the name of one of the major and minor pairs among the Six Spirit formulas in that section of the *Fǔxíngjué*.

4.5 Connecting Fives and Sixes Between Hàn and Sòng?

Another major medical innovation, which we can conclusively date to several centuries after the Hàn dynasty at the earliest, is the theory of the "Five Movements and Six Qi" (五運六氣 *wǔyùn liùqì*). In her excellent article "The System of the Five Circulatory Phases and the Six Seasonal Influences" in Elisabeth Hsu, ed., *Innovation in Chinese Medicine*, Catherine Despeux determines that it is "prudent to date its development in the field of medicine to no earlier than the eleventh century."[21] Similarly, Unschuld argues for a date of compilation for the seven "great discourses" (*dàlùn* 大論, i.e., *Sùwèn* chapters 66 through 74) of no earlier than Wáng Bīng's involvement, which means the eighth century. While these seven chapters are generally believed to have been introduced by Wáng Bīng in the eighth century, no other major medical texts of this period or earlier editions of the *Sùwèn* mention it or show its influence until the eleventh century, when it quickly became quite popular. In any case, beginning in the tenth century, medical texts discuss the prevalence of what Despeux translates as "five circulatory movements and six seasonal influences," which "gradually pervaded every field of medicine: prognosis, diagnosis, prevention, pharmacotherapy, and acupuncture."[22] This system involves the "Five Movements" (in the order of creation but starting with earth in the center: earth, metal,

[21] Catherine Despeux, "The System of the Five Circulatory Phases and the Six Seasonal Influences" in Elisabeth Hsu, ed., *Innovation in Chinese Medicine*, pp. 121–165.

[22] Ibid., p. 121.

water, wood, fire), which are here associated with five sections of the sky, identified by the twenty-eight lunar mansions traversed by the "movement" dominant or active at any particular time. These Five Movements are combined with the six Qì, as the six climatic influences, which are associated with the *wǔxíng* by subdividing Fire into "Sovereign Fire" and Ministerial Fire" and with the six Yīn-Yáng modalities in this order: Wind/Wood/Juéyīn, Fire/Sovereign Fire/Shàoyīn, Summer-Heat/Ministerial Fire/Shàoyáng, Dampness/Earth/Tàiyīn, Dryness/Metal/Yángmíng, and Cold/Water/Tàiyáng. These six Qì are subdivided into two sets of seasonal influences, the earthly "host Qì" (主氣 *zhǔqì*) and the celestial "intrusive Qì" (客氣 *kèqì*). The interaction within this complicated system of temporal and spatial modalities allows us by means of complex astrocalendrical calculations to gain time- and space-specific information for medical prognosis, diagnosis, prevention, and therapy. Despeux situates the origins of this literature and worldview in Daoist circles, in texts like the *Qǐxuánzǐ yuánhé jìyòng jīng* 啟玄子元和紀用經 from the late tenth century. Of interest to us here is the fact that this literature for the first time described the use of materia medica, previously categorized by only flavor and thermal nature, in an effort to reinforce or balance what she calls "the six yin/yang modalities" and the *wǔxíng*. Even if their precise meaning and association differed somewhat from traditional medical theories of the *wǔxíng* resonances on the one hand, and the *liùjīng* of classical formulary literature on the other, this kind of thinking strikes me as a logical progression from the information we find in the *Fǔxíngjué*, which may be one of the first text, depending on its date, to connect formula literature and medicinals with the system of *wǔxíng* resonances. In this sense, the text is clearly not an ancestor to Zhāng Zhòngjǐng's formulas and thus cannot possibly serve as a foundational text in the development of Hàn dynasty medical literature. Instead, it is important as one example of the first efforts to connect the three previously separate strands of *běncǎo* literature, formularies, and theoretical treatises, and thus as a missing link between the Hàn dynasty classics and the full-blown expression of this synthesis in Daoist-inspired texts on *wǔyùn liùqì* theory from the tenth century on. Coincidently, this is exactly the time period that Chinese medical historians suggest for the date of composition of this text.

Paul U. Unschuld addresses what he considers an unsolved puzzle to this day in the chapter on "Substance Therapy: From Materia Medica to Pharmacology" in his *Huang Di Nei Jing: Nature, Knowledge, Imagery in an Ancient Chinese Medical Text*. It is worth citing at length here because it quickly dispels some of the erroneous notions about the development of Chinese pharmaceutics between the Hàn and the Sòng dynasties that are currently held by some Western practitioners of Chinese medicine:

> *For more than a thousand years, a divide opened between a materia medica tradition virtually untouched by vessel theory and the yin-yang and five-agents doctrines of systematic correspondence, on the one hand, and an acupuncture tradition based on these very principles, on the other.... [*The Shānghánlùn*] associates the effects of therapeutic drugs with the conduits and the yin-yang doctrine. However, this remained an isolated event. Zhang Ji failed to arouse any widespread interest in his approach until the final years of the Song dynasty, when authors such as Kou Zongshi 寇宗奭 (fl. 1116) and Wang Haogu 王好古 (fl. 1246–1248) were among the first to create a pharmacology of systematic correspondence.*
>
> *Kou Zongshi, Wang Haogu, and their contemporaries of the Song-Jin-Yuan era did not have to start from zero, however. In the so-called seven comprehensive discourses of* Su wen *66 through 74, which Wang Bing added to the main text in the eighth century, no individual substances are named. Nevertheless, here is where we find much of the theoretical basis for including the application of pharmacotherapy in*

> *the doctrines of systematic correspondences.... All we can say is that they failed to influence any text of the received literature before the twelfth century, when, obviously for the first time, a pharmacology of systematic correspondence of individual substances was conceptualized.*[23]

As Unschuld and Despeux, and a host of medical historians writing in Chinese, have made eminently clear, it was one of the great innovations of the Sòng-Jīn-Yuán period that medical authors finally began to interpret the effect of medicinal substances on the body in light of vessel theory and the theory of Yīn-Yáng and *wǔxíng* resonances. Academically-minded readers are encouraged to learn about the cosmological and philosophical ruminations popular in religious and philosophical circles during the Sòng dynasty, which are strikingly relevant to this way of thinking. It is essential that we keep this historical context, and the commonly accepted facts of Chinese medical history, in mind when we try to assess the dates and relationships between the multiple distinct and unrelated textual layers in a manuscript, of which the original copy was destroyed in the mid-twentieth century and of which we only have twenty-one different memorized versions.

4.6 The Term 天行 "Celestial Movements"

To return to language as an indicator for the age of the *Fǔxíngjué* and very much related to this last observation, one term that immediately raised red flags in my mind when I first started looking closely at this text is the phrase 天行 *tiānxíng*. Literally translated, it means "movements" or "actions" (行) in or of "heaven" or the "sky." This phrase is usually equated with "epidemic" in modern

[23] Paul U. Unschuld, *Huang Di Nei Jing: Nature, Knowledge, Imagery in an Ancient Chinese Medical Text* (University of California, 2003), pp. 287–288.

translations of Chinese medicine. A digital search for this phrase in the Hàn dynasty medical texts, namely *Huángdì nèijīng, Nànjīng, Shānghánlùn,* and *Jīnguì yàolüe*, produced exactly zero hits! By contrast, when we search for this term in literature that was produced several centuries later, we find, for example, ten occurrences in the *Ishimpō* 醫心方 ("Formulas from the Heart of Medicine," a Japanese compilation of medieval Chinese medical texts from 984 CE), ten instances also in Sūn Sīmiǎo's *Bèijí qiānjīn yàofāng* from 652, four in Cháo Yuánfāng's 巢元方 *Zhūbìng yuánhòulùn* 諸病源候論 from 610, and ten in Gě Hóng's 葛洪 *Zhǒuhòu bèijífāng* 肘後備急方 ("Formulas to Prepare for Emergency to Keep up one's Sleeve," early fourth century). These findings show that "celestial movements" was clearly a popular concept in technical literature from medieval times on but, as a technical term, did not exist during the Hàn period. This is the reason why in Zhāng Zhòngjǐng's work, related pathologies in similar formulas are referred to instead as "cold damage" (傷寒 *shānghán*). In fact, medical historians in China mostly equate the term "cold damage" as used by Zhāng Zhòngjǐng with the term *tiānxíng* as used in the following centuries.[24] Instead, I read the term in the *Fǔxíngjué* literally as "celestial movements," as having a deeper significance than either the classical Chinese concept of "cold damage" or the biomedical, and later TCM, concept of "epidemics," and therefore choose to preserve its literal meaning, along the lines discussed by Sharon Weizenbaum in her commentary to Section Five on the "external contractions of celestial movements." The reason for this decision is not just poetic but because it serves as an important reminder of the significance of the actual movements in heaven and/or the sky for the physiology and pathology of the human body, in the minds of the medieval authors who embraced

[24] For an English example, see Wáng Shūmín's article cited above: "Tangye jingfa (Canonical Methods for Brews and Decoctions) 湯液經法: A Lost Text Recorded in the Hanshu Bibliography," in Vivienne Lo and Christopher Cullen, eds., *Medieval Chinese Medicine: The Dunhuang Medical Manuscripts* (Routledge, 2005), pp. 322–344.

this phrase and used it with gusto. Figures like Sūn Sīmiǎo, Gě Hóng, and Táo Hóngjǐng were all active and devoted practitioners of the arts of alchemy and spiritual and physical transformation in pursuit of longevity and immortality. They are known to have spent extended periods of time in retreat and seclusion on high mountain peaks where they were undoubtedly exposed to the elements and physically and spiritually, literally and metaphorically, much closer to, and resonating more powerfully with, "celestial movements" than most of us modern humans will ever be. As an insightful comment in the *Fǔxíngjué* credited to Táo Hóngjǐng states:

> *All those generations of students of the Dào, they pursue eternal life. But first they must get rid of illness. Regardless of whether they suffer from long-standing ailments or seasonal trouble, they must rely on the single rule of supplementing and draining the five* zàng *organs. Taking numerous preparations of medicinal formulas, they must make their* zàng Qì *balanced and harmonious, and only then may they advance to cultivate the Dào of internal visualization. Otherwise the five* jīng *Essences will not be joined, the Perfected One will be difficult to safeguard, and they will fail to enter the state of Perfection. Even though taking medicinals and getting rid of illness may be associated with trifling affairs [compared to the lofty goals of seeking immortality], it is nevertheless the core to beginning one's studies.*

Similarly, in his introduction to the six spirit and two dawning formulas, he makes this point:

> *Those of us who dwell secluded in mountains and forests are all of a sudden confronted with critical illnesses of external contraction that are difficult to avoid. With numerous transmissions and changes each day, life and death are often on the line within only three to five days. How could we possibly be careless about this! If we are able to deeply*

understand these several formulas, then we might just avoid the worrisome prospect of this risk.

What emerges from these comments that are ascribed to Táo Hóngjǐng but must have come from the brush of an anonymous author in the following centuries is that the *Fǔxíngjué* is the product of a world of practitioners dedicated deeply to physical and spiritual cultivation, with the ultimate goal of transforming their mortal bodies into immortal ones. To meet the challenges of this journey, the treatment of illness was perhaps a rudimentary and "common" step, but one that was clearly necessary as a prerequisite to the more complicated and esoteric practices that followed, once the body was in perfect working order. Likewise, Sūn Sīmiǎo also emphasizes the appropriate succession in the use of medicinal formulas on the long and arduous path to immortality:

As a great principle of taking elixirs of immortality, there always has to be a progression and order. Without knowing the technical details for these practices, not only will you suffer injury from sexual intercourse, but ultimately you will also fail to gain their power. As such, the grand rule of taking elixirs for immortality is this: First, you must get rid of the Three Worms. Once the Three Worms are gone, then you take herbal medicine. Once you have fully gained the power of this medicine, then you take tree medicine next. Once you have finished gaining its power, next you take stone medicine. Only when you rely on this succession and order will you be able to accord with the nature of these medicines, and all your different affairs will be stable and at ease, so that you can thereby extend your age![25]

This is the context in which we have to read our text and interpret its language. As such, the phrase "celestial movement" takes on an

[25] Sūn Sīmiǎo, *Bèijí qiānjīn yàofāng* volume 27 on "Nurturing the Inner Nature." See my forthcoming book on this topic.

added meaning, especially when we recall popular Daoist practices of visualization meditations like "pacing the handle and stepping on the Dipper" (步罡踏斗 *bùgāng tàdǒu*), an important and common ritual practice that involved literally stepping on each star drawn on a map of the Big Dipper and visualizing the divine inhabitants and environments of each stop. While the fine details of this journey go far beyond the limitations of this Introduction, the repeated use of the phrase "celestial movements" in what is most likely the oldest layer of the *Fǔxíngjué* does serve as yet another powerful reminder of the medieval origin of this text.

4.7 The "Six Extremes" 六極

Pointing to the same time period as the date of compilation of the *Fǔxíngjué*, another set of phrases that caught my attention during translation was the term 六極 *liùjí* , literally "six extremes," and their specific references. Like the phrase 天行 *tiānxíng* "celestial movements," this set of six different extreme pathologies is found frequently in Táng and later medical texts, but not before then! As a technical term in traditional medical literature, it refers to six different states of extreme vacuity taxation. These "six extremes" are usually listed as 氣極 *qìjí* (Qì Extreme), 血極 *xuèjí* (Blood Extreme), 筋極 *jīnjí* (Sinew Extreme), 骨極 *gǔjí* (Bone Extreme), 精極 *jīngjí* (Essence Extreme), and 髓極 *suìjí* (Marrow Extreme). The earliest record that I have found for this concept is Cháo Yuánfāng's *Zhūbìng yuánhòulùn* from 610, in the introduction to the chapter on "Vacuity Taxation," where he defines it as "Five Taxation, Six Extremes, and Seven Damages." Among these, the Six Extremes are described as follows:

> *The Six Extremes: The first is called Qì Extreme and causes the person to suffer from internal vacuity, insufficiency in the five* zàng *organs, a profusion of evil Qì and a lack of right Qì, and reluctance to speak. The*

second is called Blood Extreme and causes the person to suffer from a lack of color in the face, hair loss in the eyebrows and on the head, and mental confusion and forgetfulness. The third is called Sinew Extreme and causes the person to suffer from frequent twisted sinews, pain in all the ten finger and ten toe nails, and bitter fatigue and inability to stand for a long time. The fourth is called Bone Extreme and causes the person to suffer from soreness and whittling away, severe pain in the teeth, vexing pain in the hands and feet, inability to stand, and reluctance to move. The fifth is called Flesh Extreme and causes the person to suffer from marked emaciation, lack of moistness and luster, and failure to engender flesh and skin from food and drink. The sixth is called Essence Extreme and causes the person to suffer from shortness of breath and a droning sound, internal vacuity, insufficiency in the Qì of the five zàng *organs, loss of hair on the head, and sadness and forgetfulness.*

Similar lists, which clearly are inspired by this earliest citation, are found in slightly later medieval texts like the *Bèijí qiānjīn yàofāng*, the *Wàitái mìyào* and the *Ishimpō*. As a contemporary classically oriented practitioner of Chinese medicine, you may just have read over this concept since you have probably encountered it elsewhere. For me as a medical historian, however, it stuck out as a distinctly medieval concept that did not exist yet in the literature of the Hàn dynasty "classics."

4.8 Medieval Religious and Philosophical Terminology, Especially 體 "Substance" and 用 "Application"

In addition to the technical medical language, we also find religious and philosophical language in this text that points to an origin of at least some of the textual layers in a medieval Daoist environment: For example, the expression 真景 *zhēnjǐng*, which I have translated as "state of perfection" and which the text mentions in the introductory essay, becomes quite common beginning in the Sòng dynasty but is not found in any earlier literature. Examples like these are found throughout the text. Even the title of the text itself contains the loaded Buddhist compound 法要, literally "essentials of the Dharma" and here meaning something like "Truth" or "Principles," or in my translation "Key." This term did not exist in the Hàn dynasty.

To mention just one last pair of characters that point to a medieval date for the *Fǔxíngjué*, at the earliest, the complementary conceptual pairing of 體 *tǐ* ("substance") and 用 *yòng* ("application") requires a closer look. To begin with, however, we should clarify that these two terms are found in a chart that is one of several graphic aspects that are all or in part included in some but not all of the twenty-one different versions of the *Fǔxíngjué* submitted by Zhāng Dàchāng and his disciples, and found in different locations of the text. To refresh your memory, here is a copy of this chart:

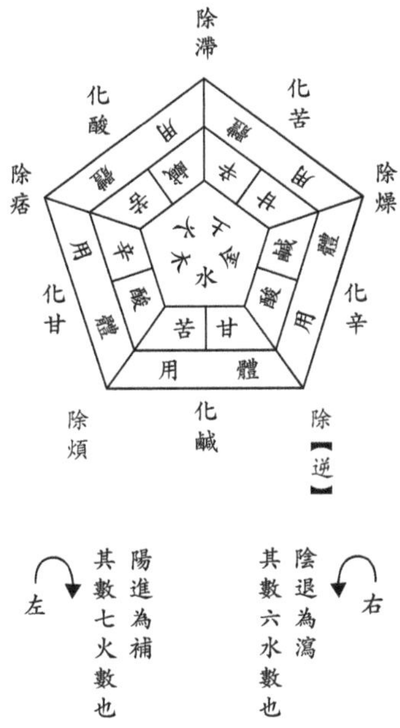

For more information on the different manuscript versions of the text, see below. Personally, I have my doubts on whether this chart was actually even part of the original Dūnhuáng manuscript, or at least its earlier layers, based on the fact that these kinds of visual representations of cosmological, medical, religious, or philosophical relations only became popular from the Sòng period on but are not found in any earlier manuscripts. I have consulted on this chart specifically with the medical historian Vivienne Lo who specializes in medical illustrations in early and medieval manuscripts, and she has confirmed my suspicions.[26] Dr. Lo is eminently familiar with this topic as the main editor, with Christopher Cullen, of *Medieval Chinese Medicine: The Dunhuang Medical Manuscripts* (RoutledgeCurzon, 2005) and, with Penelope Barrett, of the gorgeously illustrated *Imagining Chinese Medicine* (Brill, 2018). Incidentally, that book is a collection of essays and images derived from an international conference on medical illustrations that she organized with Wáng Shūmín in Běijīng in 2005 in honor of Mǎ Jìxìng's 80th birthday, where I personally got to congratulate Professor Mǎ who is one of my great heroes. In other words, if we had incontrovertible evidence that this manuscript, and the chart in particular, dated from pre-Sòng times, it would be a revolutionary finding for the history of medical illustrations in China. In light of the questionable history of this text, we may be better off treating these illustrations with a question mark. For the sake of comparison, here is a similar chart from one of the earliest texts to discuss the doctrine of the "Five Movements and Six Qì," namely the *Qǐxuánzǐ yuánhé jìyòng jīng* 啟玄子元和紀用經 from the late tenth century already mentioned above.

[26] Personal communication from October 25, 2020.

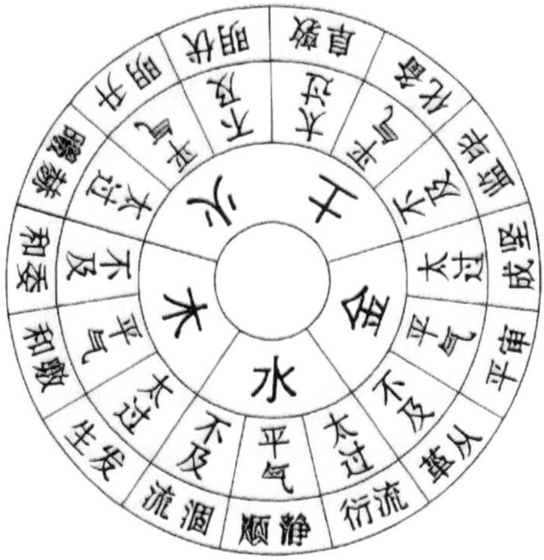

Putting aside for the moment the problems with the location and context of the chart within the content of the *Fŭxíngjué*, it is noteworthy that the juxtaposition of the concepts 體 *tĭ* ("substance") and 用 *yòng* ("application") found in the central position of each of the five pie slices in the pentagon introduces a pair of terms that the Buddhologist Charles Muller characterized as follows in an article on "The Emergence of Essence-Function 體用 Hermeneutics in the Sinification of Indic Buddhism":

> *If we can characterize the broad history of the usage and study of essence-function in East Asian thought by saying that the paradigm was first born out of the early Chinese classics, then significantly deepened in the process of its incorporation into, and transformation of, Buddhism, we can also say that it finally becomes the comprehensive matrix for Neo-Confucian philosophy, with Neo-Confucian concepts swimming around in the sea of ti-yong like fish in water. There is nothing that goes on in Neo-Confucian thought that is not either circumscribed by, or about, or spoken in reference to essence and function, or one of its narrower analogues.*[27]

[27] A. Charles Muller, "The Emergence of Essence-Function 體用 Hermeneutics in the Sinification of Indic Buddhism," in 佛教學 Review 19 (June, 2016), consulted

As he outlines in detail in this article, the pairing is already found in early philosophical discourse, such as Wáng Bì's 王弼 third-century commentary on the *Dàodéjīng* 道德經 (Classic of Dào and its Virtue/Potency). In the early philosophical literature, it is used to frame the contrast between the underlying principle or essence of things and their (temporary) human use or value, such as the discussion on 才/材 *cái* in the stories of the goose that did not honk or the gnarled useless tree in the *Zhuāngzǐ* 莊子. It was then adopted as a philosophical framework for sinicizing Buddhist perspectives beginning with Zhìyǐ 智顗 (538–597) and assuming ever greater relevance in Chán 禪 and Huáyán 華嚴 Buddhism, with such associations as sudden versus gradual enlightenment, subject versus object, or principle versus phenomenon (理-事). Eventually this juxtaposition was translated into the pair 理-氣 "Principle—Qì," which became ubiquitous in Neo-Confucian discourse, especially in the writings of Zhū Xī 朱熹 (1130–1200).

What needs to concern us here in the context of the *Fǔxíngjué* is merely its presence in this chart, which we can interpret in a number of different ways. Given the popularity of this juxtaposition in religious and philosophical discourse beginning in the sixth century, but in particular during the Sòng dynasty, it strongly points to a later date for the text within the generally accepted range of sixth through tenth centuries. Alternatively, we could argue that it merely suggests that the chart may have been a later addition. A third possibility is, perhaps unintentionally and I would argue most likely mistakenly, evident in Wáng Shūmín's English article "*Tangye jingfa* 湯液經法: A lost text recorded in the *Hanshu* bibliography," which I have discussed above. It is not impossible that this last reading of these two terms in the pentagonal chart was actually introduced not by Prof. Wáng but during the process of translating her article into English and pre-

online at http://www.acmuller.net/articles/2016-06-tiyong-critical-review.pdf

paring it for publication. Let me explain: In the English version of the chart, as depicted on p. 332 of that publication, the five "dynamic agents" or "elements" (wood, fire, earth, metal, and water) are not placed in the central inner-most section of each of the five pie charts, but instead in the middle of each slice, right between the characters 用 (application) and 體 (substance), with no vertical line in between. As most of the hand-drawn versions of the chart among the various manuscripts submitted by Zhāng Dàchāng and his disciples show, the consensus in their reading of this chart was definitely that these characters described the two flavors in the outgoing spokes of each pie slice associated with the "element" or "dynamic agent" of that slice. So for example, in the case of wood, the "application" 用 is acrid and the "substance" 體 is sour. Reading the three characters in one line as 用木體, however, Wáng Shūmín, or possibly her English translator who has not seen other versions of this pentagonal chart, render this as a sentence and translate it as "embodiment through wood," followed by "embodiment through fire," "embodiment through earth," and so on. It is pretty clear to me that this is either a mistranslation into English, or alternatively a way for Wáng Shūmín to avoid the juxtaposition of 體 and 用, which strongly suggests a date for the text many centuries later than as a citation of the *Tāngyèjīng* from the Hàn dynasty. This reading of the phrase is highly unlikely given the fact that most depictions of the chart do place the "element/dynamic agent" 行 on its own in the innermost section of each of the five pie slices and that the chart carries, for example, the following lengthy title in at least one version by Liú Déxìng 劉德興 from 1974: "Chart for matching the ruler, minister, assistants, and envoys, supplementing and draining, substance and application, and changes in the essential methods for using medicinals for the five *zàng* organs." So we are left with yet another strong argument for dating at least that layer of the *Fǔxíngjué* to the sixth century at the earliest, but most likely several centuries later when the religious use of this conceptual pair had made its way into other forms of discourse.

5

The Different Manuscript Versions

One last question to address in this Introduction to the *Fǔxíngjué*, which some of the arguments above have already touched on, is the existence of twenty-one different manuscript versions of the text. As described above, all of these versions were written down by Zhāng Dàchāng and his disciples on the basis of Zhāng's memory of the original, which, he claims, had been obtained by his grandfather in the early twentieth century and was then destroyed during the Cultural Revolution. The present book is not the place to go into detail on this topic, and I generally have chosen to just follow the lead of the medical historians in China who have researched this issue for many years with great care and skill. Nevertheless, it is helpful to touch on some points in the following paragraphs, to give the reader a general impression of the differences and similarities.

To begin with, let us look at the already-mentioned controversy around illustrations. The only graphic element included in the critical editions published by medical historians — as opposed to Chinese publications of the text by clinical authors from among Zhāng's disciples, who lack the necessary training to determine historical accuracy — is the pentagonal chart that associates each of the *wǔxíng* in five pie slices with the two flavors associated with "substance" 體 and "application" 用, the flavor that it transforms 化, and the pathology that it eliminates 除. In some manuscript versions, this chart is placed at the very beginning of the text, in others in the middle between the formulas for supplementing and draining the five *zàng* organs and the formulas for external contraction of celestial movements, and in some at the end. Most manuscripts leave the chart without a title.

Many of the manuscripts, including all of the earlier versions, have two additional charts, in the form of two tables that list the main ingredients used for supplementing and draining the five *zàng* organs in their roles as rulers, ministers, and assistants and envoys. The earliest manuscript that exists, for example, is the version from 1965 by Fàn Zhìliáng 范志良, which is a reconstruction based on Fàn's notes from Zhāng Dàchāng's teaching. It contains two tables that are inserted between the first two sections of the text, or in other words between Section One on "Differentiating Patterns of *Zàng* Organ Disease" and Section Two on "Five Formulas to Address Drainage of the Five *Zàng* Organs." These two tables are preceded by a line stating: "To summarize the method of using medicinals in the Minor Supplementing and Draining Decoctions for the Five *Zàng* Organs, here is attached a table to the left." The tables themselves are titled "Using Medicinals for Supplementation" and "Using Medicinals for Draining," respectively. These same two tables, with slightly different names, plus a third one that categorizes the twenty-five medicinals in columns and rows associated with the *wǔxíng*, are also found in Zhāng Dàchāng's first submitted manuscript from 1974, but are there placed right after the pentagonal chart that is the only illustration to have made it into any critical published editions of the text. Complicating matters, Táo Hóngjǐng's comment ("This chart indeed [reflects] the utterly significant subtlety of the classical methods of decoctions. When those who study them are able to know them by heart, their Dào of medicine has reached its destination!"), which in the standard published edition thus seems to refer clearly to the pentagonal chart, looks in other editions from its placement AFTER the pentagonal chart to refer to the other illustrations.

Incidentally, Zhāng Dàchāng's first version is missing the whole part of the *Fǔxíngjué* that follows after the chart, namely Section Five on "Classical Treatments for External Contraction," or in other words the Two Dawn and Six Spirit formulas and the "Emergency

Treatments for Opening the Orifices"! This omission forces us once again to reconsider one of the arguments cited by modern proponents for reading that section, or by extension the entire *Fǔxíngjué*, as a Hàn dynasty text and as equivalent to the *Tāngyèjīng*.

In addition, there is a whole other set of substantial information found in many, but not all, of the manuscripts that is not included in the printed critical editions or, for that reason, in my own translation. That section offers formulas, charts, and commentary by Táo Hóngjǐng or his impersonator, pertaining to the medicinal use of mineral substances, parallel to the sections on herbal ingredients. We find:

- tables that display five-fold sets of minerals associated with supplementing and draining the five *zàng* organs,
- lists of minerals categorized by the five flavors and then subcategorized by the *wǔxíng*,
- lists of minerals as treatments for taxation of the five *zàng* organs,
- sets of major and minor "powder decoction methods" for supplementing and draining each of the five *zàng* organs, and additional commentary.

The absence of this information from the major published critical editions of the *Fǔxíngjué* in Chinese, such as the collections of Dūnhuáng medical manuscripts edited by Mǎ Jìxìng and Cóng Chūnyǔ, demonstrates that the editors in charge of these publications deemed only one of the charts worthy of inclusion but must have considered the other charts, as well as the material on minerals, modern additions and therefore left them out. No reasons are given for these major editorial decisions.

Unfortunately, these important details are invisible to modern readers who are only looking at a single printed edition or, worse yet in the case of Western students, receive the transmission in PowerPoint slides or handouts that never introduce the text as a whole in its original form and structure at all but rearrange it in excerpts. I will spare the reader a detailed examination and cross-comparison of all twenty-one versions of the *Fǔxíngjué* and trust that the critical editions published by such authorities as Mǎ Jīxìng and Cóng Chūnyǔ are the result of many years of painstaking comparative research, which these scholars are much better equipped to perform than any of us. As such, the main source text for my own critical edition and translation was the published version in Cóng Chúnyǔ 叢春雨, lead editor, *Dūnhuáng zhōngyīyào quánshū* 敦煌中醫藥全書 (Zhongyi guji chubanshe, 1994), which is in turn based on the version of the text memorized and recorded by Zhāng Dàchāng 張大昌, supplemented with the versions memorized by his disciples.

6

Conclusion

Can you now see how the multiple copies and versions and transmissions of this text introduce layer upon layer upon layer of confusion, uncertainty, and yet more misinterpretations? While this complicated textual history has caused my brain to do somersaults in this past year of working with the *Fǔxíngjué*, it does not have to be of immediate concern to you, dear reader, if you are only interested in the clinical relevance of the content.

The most important insight that I do want to share with you is that we are dealing with multiple versions of an unstable text, often differing substantially in structure, order of information, and even content, all of which were reconstructed from memory during a tumultuous time in Chinese history on the basis of a single man's recollections of a manuscript supposedly acquired by his grandfather from a mysterious monk in a far-away place in the early twentieth century. There is no way to prove at this point which parts of these reconstructions, if any, were additions by Zhāng Dàchāng or his disciples and which were "authentic," and even what "authentic" may mean in this case. Given the work done by Chinese medical historians on this text, I follow their lead in what I consider the "authentic" layers, order, and content of the text and use their critical editions as the source text for my own translation. Also following their lead, I consider this "authentic" core of the text to be an anonymously compiled manuscript consisting of multiple textual layers from the sixth through tenth centuries, which was stored, sealed, and preserved in the Library Cave in Dūnhuáng until discovered in the beginning of the twentieth century. This text contains what appears to be a group of formulas, namely the Two Dawning and Six Spirit Formulas that strike us modern readers as "classical," in the sense of harking back to the Hàn dynasty, because of their name, structure, ingredients, and similarity to some of Zhāng Zhòngjǐng's formulas. It is impossible to reconstruct at this point whether Zhāng Zhòngjǐng's work and this layer of the *Fǔxíngjué* share a third text as a common ancestor, or whether this part of the *Fǔxíngjué* was intentionally created many centuries after Zhāng Zhòngjǐng's lifetime on the basis of classical formulas, to appear more ancient than the rest of the text. The main message I want you to take away from this whole lengthy introduction is that we are looking at a fascinating medieval text with a complicated history but precious content, significant for both medical historians and contemporary clinicians. While possibly containing earlier elements, the text as a whole cannot possibly date to the Hàn dynasty, and we must therefore be careful not to read or interpret it as such. I leave it up to you, dear reader, to determine for yourself the clinical usefulness of the material that follows. Suffice it to say that I would not have gone through the trouble of publishing an entire book on the *Fǔxíngjué*, or bothered my busy colleague Sharon Weizenbaum to contribute clinical commentary, if I didn't see any concrete value for contemporary practitioners of Chinese medicine in this material. I do sincerely hope that you will find the following information helpful in alleviating the suffering of your patients, since that is what all of our shared work is ultimately all about.

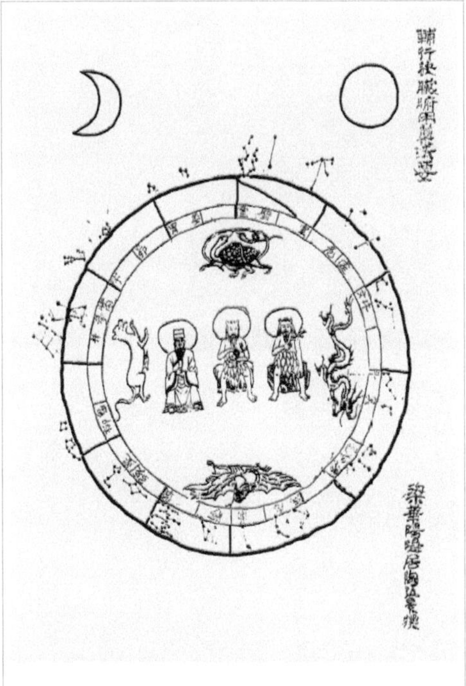

《辅行诀》卷首“三皇四神二十八宿星图”（王子旭提供，王秉灿画师手绘）

This image comes from the cover of one of the manuscript versions of the *Fǔxíngjué*, by Wáng Zǐxù 王子旭 from 1964. It is included in Zhāng Dàchāng 張大昌 and Qián Chāochén 錢超塵, *Fǔxíngjué wǔzàng yòngyào fǎyào chuánchéngjí* 《辅行诀五臟用药法要》傳承集 (Collected Transmissions of *Fǔxíngjué wǔzàng yòngyào fǎyào*), Xuéyuàn chūbǎnshè 學苑出版社, 2008. p. 5.

Acknowledgments

Written mostly during the great lockdown of 2020 due to the Covid-19 pandemic, not a day has passed in the creation of this book when I have not been reminded of the importance of appreciating "celestial movements" at this time of profound change, challenge, and potential. At this very moment, (early December, 2020), many humans are struggling with adjusting to the current "celestial movements" and they are actually making it difficult for me to write what is usually my favorite piece of any book I publish, namely these acknowledgments. But perhaps the challenging celestial environment is simply a gentle reminder to think a little harder, dig a little deeper, and feel a little more strongly into that deep well of gratitude that is always the inexhaustible source for each of my books.

So let us start with this unfathomable yet inexhaustible wellspring, the headwater of this project. Translating this image into a search for the misty origins of the present book, my ultimate source of inspiration for writing is always the ancient literature, for the traces of the deep wisdom that I find expressed there. Like the pure white snow on the distant peaks that mysteriously feeds the mountain spring emerging seemingly from nowhere between the rocks under my feet, such terms as "celestial movements" (天行 *tiānxíng*) or "state of perfection" (真景 *zhēnjǐng*, or alternatively "scenery of truth," "landscape of the genuine," "authentic condition of embodied actualization"), in my highly inadequate English rendering, are what tickle my fancy and get me going. Classics like the *Dàodéjīng* 道德經 (Classic of the Dào and its Virtue-Power), the *Yìjīng* 易經 (Classic of Changes) or the *Huángdì nèijīng* 黃帝內經 (Yellow Emperor's Inner Classic) are my pure mountain snow, which I return to again and again for a taste of that blissful state that the Yellow Emperor's Classic refers to as 清靜 *qīngjìng* "purity and stillness." It is the great irony of my life that my path to this stillness runs through what seems its very opposite, the loud exhausting computer-based "busy-ness" of publishing, in the literal sense of making something public. Yet, from the stillness of the mountain top we shall eventually arrive at the stillness of the unending ocean, I hope....

Since we have all been stuck at home now for close to a year, unable to travel, we may as well engage in a flight of fancy together. Let us pursue the tiny trickle of the original headwater spring down from a remote mountain crevice all the way to the sea. Along the way, we first get to traverse lush flower meadows before we shall joyously tumble into still collecting pools of radiant turquoise snowmelt. For this book, in addition to the classical headwater on high, the other main source feeding the original trickle has been the painstaking research of historians and philologists in the broad field of "traditional Chinese medicine," many personal teachers and friends, who have laid the foundations that made my own work possible. You will find the names of most of them in the Preface and References sections. Among them, Christopher Cullen, Cathérine Despeux, Charlotte Furth, Marta Hanson, Donald Harper, Elisabeth Hsu, Lǐ Jiànmín, Vivienne Lo, Mǎ Jìxìng, Mayanagi Makoto, Wáng Shūmín, Paul U. Unschuld, and Yi-Li Wu are just some of the academics who have shaped my own way of thinking, my ability to critically read classical Chinese medical literature, and my line of questioning. This book has reminded me in a very tangible way what a debt of gratitude I owe to their work and to my academic training. My own research into the *Fǔxíngjué* is but a small and inadequate taste of their scholarship, hopefully presented in a way that makes this important field of academic inquiry enticing for our clinical colleagues.

To return to the metaphor of the stream of knowledge descending from its lofty but lonely mountain peaks, let us rest for a moment in the pristine cold alpine pools that slowed and at the same time enriched my creative flow. Gathering the various streams of philosophy, medicine, cosmology, poetry and uncategorizable teachings, to overflow into one larger outlet when the time was ripe, were perhaps the countless conversations I have been having over the past decades with my clinical colleagues. Dear friends like Deirdre Courtney (whose Irish whiskey heats me up after wintry ocean swims), Z'ev Rosenberg (whose questions keep me on my toes), Debra Betts (whose special possum wool socks keep my feet warm during long cold days of writing), Paul Magarelli (whose biomedical perspective on my classical teachings is more tantalizing than rhubarb pie), and so many others have enthusiastically embraced the many chances to stew with me over the relationship between the macrocosm and the microcosm of the human body. This past year, the opportunities for creative cross-fertilization at international conferences like the annual TCM Congress in Rothenburg, Germany or the Integrative Fertility Symposium up in Vancouver, Canada were dearly missed, but the lack of travel meant more undisturbed writing time for me. Furthermore, innovative Zoom offerings like the Pacific Symposium or Eastern Currents' *Net of Knowledge*, in addition to books and journals and the many thoughtful conversations I have so enjoyed hosting in the framework of my own "Tea Time Talks"[1] have all fed my pool in ways that I could have never imagined a year ago.

I owe a particular debt of gratitude to three colleagues for this book project: More than anybody else, Sharon Weizenbaum helped me

[1] See https://www.imperialtutor.com/teatimetalks for more information.

to clarify the direction, importance, and final shape of this book. By providing a Foreword and an extensive clinical commentary on what may be the earliest layer of the text, namely the formulas for "external contractions of celestial movements" in Section Five, Sharon has enriched this book by making it more directly clinically applicable. In addition, my understanding of Chinese medicine has benefited immensely from her gracious gesture of welcoming me into her outstanding Graduate Mentorship. Our conversations about the importance of reading this book critically in its appropriate historical context were such great fun and mutually enlightening that our poor farm animals on both ends of the Zoom calls often had to wait for their meals or milking. But at least our roosters learned to greet each other through the computer! I only hope our collaboration will continue beyond this project and may perhaps inspire others to engage in similar projects that bridge the chasm between academic and clinical work. In addition, her White Pine Circle has provided a new home for my Imperial Tutor mentorship that we are both looking forward to nurturing and exploring as an innovative platform for fertile exchanges of clinical and academic information. The other clinician who has cheered me on through a number of dry patches by providing feedback (and never-ending enthusiasm) based on his sensitivity for the pulse of the profession was Michael Max. His *Qiological* podcast and many class offerings are a true gift to the profession by providing a community voice at a time when meeting in person has become impossible. Definitely not last, my former colleague at the National University of Natural Medicine and heart sister Brenda Hood, who is still the smartest woman I know and most powerful practitioner ever to sink a needle into me, never fails to get my creative juices going. Her limitless curiosity, deep knowledge, bottomless heart, and passion for and humility towards this great tradition that we both get to work in are the perfect manifestation of the ideal of "life-long learning" that is an absolute must for any medical practitioner, no matter what paradigm you follow.

The stream that eventually emerges from the overflowing snowmelt pond now gradually descends into the thickly shaded world of nourishing forest. Here, we temporarily rest in shady bogs of murky rainwater, blackened by eons of decomposing leaves, fallen from above but ultimately containing the wealth of the soil pulled up from deep deep below by the roots of the ancient old-growth trees. The equivalent fertilization that this book project received at this stage would be the bottomless support and love from my family, fed in turn by all of our ancestral roots. Throughout these past few challenging months, my parents in particular have been a fountain of good cheer, patience, material and emotional support, and positive attitude, in spite of the fact that at their age a lost year without seeing their distant children and grandchildren must feel like an eternity. It is so clear to me that the unimaginable suffering that their generation experienced during the Second World War has given them a perspective that they have been able to draw on, consciously or not, to now offer support to so many people less fortunate than they are. This has in turn inspired my daughter and me to aim to do the same. My daughter Momo Wilms-Crowe's radiant activism and passion for social justice, from prison work to houselessness to immigration support to youth education to community gardens, reminds me every day that we all can and must live our "Golden Path" (in Lillian Bridges' terms), or express our "Heavenly Destiny," our *mìng* 命, to create the world we want to live in. And in this deep mulchy forest pool of nourishment, I also include, as in every book, my dear, dear wise sister, friend, and guide, Lillian Pearl Bridges, who never fails to remind me of what truly matters in Chinese medicine. Without her encouragement, delicious dumplings, and loving phone calls, I certainly would not embrace my quirkiness with the gusto that I do or have found the strength to finish this final stretch of the marathon of this book project. More than anything, thank you for supporting my love of goats and cold ocean swims, as weird as both of those are!

As our mountain stream leaves the protective shade of the forest and enters the open plains, it is time to acknowledge some of the innumerable rivulets and brooks, tributaries and confluences that have helped it to swell into a mighty river of knowledge. Staying with this image, this is my opportunity to name the various people who have written endorsements for this book, each of whom have contributed in their own way to its creation. Many of them have also provided essential feedback and corrections along the way. Of course all errors that remain rest solely on my shoulders. In addition to the scholars and friends already mentioned above, Steve Clavey and Pierce Salguero deserve all of our gratitude as the publisher and editor-in-chief of two leading journals in the field of Chinese medicine, *The Lantern* and *Asian Medicine*, respectively. In the vein of these two journals, it is my hope that this book is a small contribution to the "meta-disciplinary approach" proposed by Dr. Salguero as the contentious yet fertile space where different paradigms rub against each other, forcing all participants to question their previously held beliefs in a shared desire to advance our understanding of Chinese medicine, with the ultimate goal of alleviating suffering. Leo Lok, Claudia Citkovitz, and Eran Even have supported this project by cheering me on and reminding me of its clinical value, which is a true honor, coming from such outstanding clinicians and thinkers! As the two amazing "wonder women" behind the Shen Nong Society with its outstanding annual conference, Caroline Radice and Sally Rappeport have created a dynamic platform for a high-level exchange of knowledge on traditional Chinese medicinal therapy. This delicious fruit of their collaboration has furthered the teaching of a *jīngfāng* style of Chinese medicine more than any other teachers, institution, or organization in the West. Their support of this project means so much to me, and I only hope that my publications in turn might support their efforts. Last but certainly not least, I want to acknowledge Robert Hoffman and Phil Settles not only for their work as practitioners and researchers but more importantly for their tireless dedication to education, as the deans of two outstanding clinical doctorate programs at Yo San University of Traditional Chinese Medicine and the Academy of Chinese Culture and Health Sciences, respectively. With their choice of diverse high-quality faculty and insistence on teaching critical thinking and solid research skills, I see them continuing the important work of my own teachers and clinical colleagues, by planting the seeds for professional growth in the next generation. Two other educational institutions whose role in contributing to my "river of knowledge" I need to mention are the Oregon College of Oriental Medicine and its close neighbor, the National University of Natural Medicine. Without knowing me personally, the librarian at OCOM was kind enough to mail me a rare Chinese book from their outstanding collection of medical texts that was crucial to my research. More importantly, she even kindly granted me several extensions on the due date. Writing on a small island in the middle of a pandemic, this sort of generous assistance among professional colleagues was very much appreciated! Lastly, the College of Classical Chinese Medicine at the National University of Natural Medicine was one of the original training grounds for my efforts at transmitting the wisdom from the classics to beginning students of Chinese medicine. Especially the Classical Texts committee, which I chaired for several years and which was central to the clinical doctorate program, proved to be a wonderful opportunity for professional exchange and clarification on the purpose, vision, limitations, and challenges of teaching classical Chinese language and medical literature as part of a demanding clinical program. I am greatly indebted to all my former colleagues at NUNM, but particularly to the members of that committee: Brenda Hood, Long Rihui, Jim Cleaver, and Joon-Hee Lee.

Returning to our river of knowledge metaphor, we now cross some long dry desert stretches but also pass by bustling cities crowded with barges and ferries, congestion and bridges, human tears and laughter, and music and art and play. This is where I find myself thinking of all the fruitful and heart-warming, inspiring and occasionally challenging interactions with students, as a visiting professor in doctoral programs, in weekend retreats, during intense conference lectures and the socializing afterwards, and of course in the framework of my Imperial Tutor mentorship program. My students' questions, gestures of appreciation, and responses, both negative and positive, have sharpened my sensitivity to the clinical application and practical meaning of what I find in my brain and heart. In this year in particular, where we have all missed out on much of this kind of interaction, I have truly learned to appreciate how nourishing the in-person transmission of knowledge is for me as the teacher. I cannot wait to gather with all of you again around a conference table, over soup pots in a retreat kitchen, kicking my shoes off at the evening dance party, or savoring those quiet moments with a cup of tea by the beach, pondering somebody's capstone project as a brilliant expression of their professional growth. More than anything else, the joy and honor of working with students of this medicine, the beautiful healers of today and tomorrow, is what keeps me going, even in the lonely work of writing a book like this.

Getting very close to reaching the final destination of our river, in a place where fresh and salt waters mix and where progress is affected by the irresistible push and pull of the tides, the construction of some straight-edged canals and the dredging of some channels for navigation have been essential, to facilitate expedient progress and avoid getting stuck in the muck. While not the most poetic or fun part of the journey, without this assistance and active intervention, there would certainly be no book in your hands. On the other hand, we can perhaps think of this last stage as the fertile estuaries, the last contact with land, before the river dissolves into the limitless sea and disappears beyond the horizon, like Laozi at the Western frontier. The equivalent in publishing to this final and ever so essential step is the exhausting work of manuscript preparation. Here I have once again been so very fortunate to have two exceptional assistants by my side: Chris Flanagan has provided invaluable proofreading and copyediting assistance, with a sensitivity to the project as a whole and to the classical medical language and concepts that no other professional editor could ever match. Following right behind, Barbara Tada has patiently worked with me through the many and often unforeseen challenges of laying out yet another book with multiple levels of text, translation, and commentary in Chinese and English. While the layout of the inside of the book is clean and crisp as always with her work, she has outdone herself again with the design of the cover. Incidentally, the gorgeous cover photograph was taken by her husband, Hidenori Tada, whose contribution I gratefully acknowledge here as well.

I thank the universe for all the blessings that have flown into this stream to make it possible for this book to appear under such challenging circumstances!

Sabine Wilms, December 9, 2020
Whidbey Island

《輔行訣臟腑用藥法要》

FǓXÍNGJUÉ ZÀNGFǓ YÒNGYÀO FǍYÀO

SECRET TIPS FOR HELPFUL ACTION: THE KEY TO USING MEDICINALS ON THE *ZÀNGFǓ* ORGANS

梁·華陽隱居 陶弘景撰

Compiled by Táo Hóngjǐng, hermit from Huáyáng, during the Liáng dynasty

Section One

Differentiating Patterns of *Zàng* Organ Disease

1.1

Introductory Essay

隱居曰：凡學道輩，欲求永年，先須祛疾。或有夙痼，或患時恙，一依五臟補瀉法例，服藥數劑，必使臟氣平和，乃可進修內視之道。不爾，五精不續，真一難守，不入真景也。

服藥祛疾，雖繫微事，亦初學之要領也。諸凡雜病，服藥汗吐下後，邪氣雖平，精氣被奪，致令五臟虛疲，當即據證服補湯數劑以補之。不然，時日久曠，或變為損證，則生死轉側耳。謹將五臟虛實證候悉列於下，庶幾識別無誤焉。

The hermit [Táo Hóngjǐng] states: All those generations of students of the Dào, they pursue eternal life. But first they must get rid of illness. Regardless of whether they suffer from long-standing ailments or seasonal trouble, they must rely on the single rule of supplementing and draining the five *zàng* organs. Taking numerous preparations of medicinal formulas, they must make their *zàng* Qì balanced and harmonious, and only then may they advance to cultivate the Dào of internal visualization. Otherwise the five *jīng* Essences will not be joined, the Perfected One will be difficult to safeguard, and they will fail to enter the state of Perfection.

Even though taking medicinals and getting rid of illness may be associated with trifling affairs [compared to the lofty goals of seeking immortality], it is nevertheless the core to beginning one's studies. For all the various illnesses, after you have taken medicine to induce sweating, vomiting, or downward discharge, even though the evil Qì has been balanced, the *jīng* Essence Qì has been carried off as well. This has caused the five *zàng* organs to be vacuous and exhausted, so that you must now take several preparations of supplementing decoctions in accordance with the pattern, to supplement them. Otherwise they will be laid waste over time or the situation will transform into a pattern of true detriment, with the eventual result of life being replaced with death! Vigilantly take the signs and symptoms of vacuity and repletion in the five *zàng* organs that are listed comprehensively below, so that you may be able to discriminate between them and make no mistakes.

Translator's Note

Regarding Táo Hóngjǐng's role in the creation and transmission of this text, the reader is asked to carefully review the pertinent information in the historical introduction of the present book. Section 2.5 of the Preface discusses Táo Hóngjǐng's potential involvement with the *Fǔxíngjué* and the problems with crediting him with the authorship of the text as a whole as well as of the statements claimed to be by him that are interspersed throughout the text. The current consensus by all the academic experts on early Chinese medical literature, many of whom have studied and written about this text extensively, most notably Mǎ Jīxìng 馬繼興, Wáng Shūmín 王淑民, and Cóng Chúnyǔ 叢春雨, place the date for the original text in the medieval period, between Táo Hóngjǐng's lifetime (456–536) and the beginning of the Sòng period in the tenth century. As such, we cannot accept these statements in the text as fact but must suspect that Táo's name was added by a later writer in order to give the text credibility and prestige.

1.2

Differentiating Patterns of Liver Disease: Essay and Formulas

辨肝臟病證文並方

肝虛則恐，實則怒。

肝病者，必兩脅下痛，痛引少腹。虛則目䀮䀮無所見，耳有所聞，心澹澹然如人將捕之。氣逆則耳聾、頰腫，治之取厥陰、少陽血者。

邪在肝，則兩脅中痛。中寒，惡血在內，則胻善瘈，節時腫。取之行間以引脅下，補三里以溫中，取耳間青脈，以去其瘈。

Vacuity in the liver results in fear. Repletion results in anger.

Illness of the liver invariably manifests with pain below both rib-sides and pain stretching into the lower abdomen. Vacuity results in blurred vision or inability to see, inability to hear, and a turbulent feeling in the heart as if somebody were about to seize them. Countercurrent movement of Qì results in deafness and swelling of the cheeks. To treat this, choose Juéyīn and Shàoyáng, drawing blood.

The presence of evil in the liver results in pain in both rib-sides. Cold strike or malign blood inside results in tendency to spasms and swelling at regular intervals in the calves. Capture it at Xíngjiān (LV-2) for the pulling [pain] below the rib-sides, supplement at the Sānlǐ points (LI-10 and ST-36) to warm the center, and choose the green-blue vessels in the area of the ears to get rid of the patient's spasms.

Translator's Note

This passage is a compilation of quotations from the *Huángdì nèijīng* 《黃帝內經》:

Língshū 《靈樞》 8:
肝藏血，血舍魂。肝氣虛則恐，實則怒。

The liver stores the blood, and the blood houses the hún *soul. Vacuity of liver Qì results in fear; repletion results in anger.*

Sùwèn 《素問》 22:

肝病者，兩脅下痛引少腹，令人善怒，虛則目𥆧𥆧無所見，耳無所聞，善恐如人將捕之，取其經，厥陰與少陽。氣逆，則頭痛，耳聾不聰，頰腫。取血者。

Illness of the liver invariably manifests with pain below both rib-sides pulling into the lower abdomen, causing a tendency to anger in the person. Vacuity results in blurred vision or inability to see, inability to hear, and a tendency to fear as if somebody were about to seize them. Choose its channels: Juéyīn and Shàoyáng. When its Qì moves countercurrent, the result is headache, deafness and lack of hearing, and swelling in the cheeks. Draw blood.

Língshū 《靈樞》 20:

邪在肝，則兩脅中痛，寒中，惡血在內，胻善掣，節時腳腫。取之行間以引脅下，補三里以溫胃中，取血脈以散惡血，取耳間青脈，以去其掣。

When the evil is in the liver, the result is pain inside both rib-sides, cold in the center, malign blood on the inside, a tendency to spasms in the calves, and swelling in the feet at regular intervals. Capture it at Xíngjiān (LV-2) in order [treat the] pulling below the rib-sides. Supplement the Sānlǐ points (LI-10 and ST-36) to warm the center of the stomach. Choose the blood vessels to disperse the malign blood and choose the green-blue vessels in the area of the ears to get rid of the patient's spasms.

In addition, a note is in order on the term "capture," which is my translation for the Chinese character 取 *qǔ*. While literally meaning "to take" or "to seize," it is often used in early medical literature to the act of "selecting" a specific point or channel for treatment with acupuncture or moxibustion. While the sense of "selecting" a certain channel for treatment would make the text more digestible to the modern reader, the presence of the direct object 之 *zhī* in the Chinese original indicates that the author did indeed mean to tell the reader to "capture it" at a certain location. I interpret this "it" as referring to the evil, in the sense that you are able to catch the evil by accessing the body for treatment via needling or burning moxa at this point.

陶云：肝德在散。故經云以辛補之，以酸瀉之。肝苦急，急食甘以緩之。適其性而衰也。

Táo [Hóngjǐng] states: The special power of the liver lies in dispersing. Therefore, the Classic says to use the acrid flavor to supplement it and the sour flavor to drain it. When the liver suffers from tension, urgently consume sweet substances to slacken it. This is a case of weakening it by conforming to its nature.

Translator's Note

This quotation from the "Classic" refers to *Sùwèn* 《素問》 22:

肝欲散，急食辛以散之，用辛補之，酸瀉之。
…肝苦急，急食甘以緩之。

The liver likes dispersing. Urgently consume acrid [substances] to disperse it. Use acrid [substances to supplement it and sour substances to drain it.... When the liver suffers from tension, urgently consume sweet [substances] to relax it.

小瀉肝湯

治肝實，兩脅下痛，痛引少腹迫急者方：

枳實（熬）	
芍藥	
生薑	各三兩

上三味，以清漿三升，煮取一升，頓服之。不瘥，即重作服之。

Xiǎo Xiè Gān Tāng
(Minor Liver-Draining Decoction)

A formula to treat liver repletion with pain below both rib-sides and pain stretching to the lower abdomen that is acute:

zhǐshí (slowly toasted)	
sháoyào	
shēngjiāng	3 *liǎng* each

Decoct the three ingredients above in 3 *shēng* of clear fermented rice water until reduced to 1 *shēng*. Quaff in a single dose. If there is no recovery, make it again and take that.

大瀉肝湯

治頭痛、目赤、多恚怒、脅下支滿而痛，痛連少腹迫急無奈方：

枳實（熬）	
芍藥	
甘草（炙）	
黃芩	
大黃	
生薑（切）	各一兩

上六味，以水五升，煮取二升，溫分再服。

Dà Xiè Gān Tāng
(Major Liver-Draining Decoction)

A formula to treat headache, redness in the eyes, profuse rage and anger, propping fullness and pain below the rib-sides, and pain connecting to the lower abdomen that is acute and unbearable:

zhǐshí (slowly toasted)	
sháoyào	
gāncǎo (mix-fried)	
huángqín	
dàhuáng	
shēngjiāng (chopped)	1 *liǎng* each

Decoct the six ingredients above in 5 *shēng* of water until reduced to 2 *shēng*. Take it warm, divided into two doses.

Translator's Note

You may want to compare this to the formula for Xiè Gān Tāng (Liver-Draining Decoction, with no distinction between "Major" and "minor") in the *Wàitái mìyào* 《外台秘藥》:

深師療肝氣實，目赤若黄，脅下急，
小便難，瀉肝湯方：
人参 甘草各三兩，炙 生薑五兩 黄芩二兩 半夏一升，
洗 大棗十四枚，擘。

右六味，切，以水五升煮半夏三、四沸，内藥，最後内薑，煎取二升，去滓，分為二服，羸人三服。忌海藻、菘菜、羊肉、餳。

Master Shēn's formula for Liver-Draining Decoction, to cure liver Qì repletion with red or yellow eyes, tension below the rib-sides, and difficult urination:

rénshēn and gāncǎo, 3 liǎng *each; mix-fried shēngjiāng* 5 liǎng*; huángqín* 2 liǎng*; bànxià* 1 shēng, *washed; dàzǎo* 14 *pieces, split.*

Take the six ingredients to the right and chop them. Decoct the bànxià in 5 shēng *of water, bringing it to a boil three or four times. Add the other herbs, with the shēngjiāng added last, and simmer until reduced to* 2 shēng. *Remove the dregs and divide and take as two doses. For an emaciated person, divide and take in three doses. Avoid hǎizǎo, bak choy cabbage, mutton, and malt sugar.*

小補肝湯

治心中恐疑，時多惡夢，氣上衝心，越汗出，頭目眩暈者方：

桂枝	
乾薑	
五味子	各三兩
棗（去核，一方作薯蕷，當從）	十二枚

上四味，以水八升，煮取三升，溫服一升，日三服。

- 心中悸者，加桂枝一兩半；
- 衝气盛者，加五味子一兩半；
- 頭若眩者，加白朮一兩半；
- 乾嘔者，去大棗，加生薑一兩半；
- 中滿者，去棗；
- 心中如飢者，還用棗；
- 咳逆頭苦痛者，加細辛一兩半；
- 四肢冷，小便難者，加附子一枚，炮。

Xiǎo Bǔ Gān Tāng
(Minor Liver-Supplementing Decoction)

A formula to treat fear and doubt in the heart, periodic profusion of malign dreams, Qì ascending to surge against the heart, intense sweating, and dizzy head and vision:

guìzhī	
gānjiāng	
wǔwèizǐ	3 *liǎng* each
dàzǎo (pitted. An alternate [version of this] formula calls for shǔyù instead. Follow that!)	12 pieces

Decoct the four ingredients above in 8 *shēng* of water until reduced to 3 *shēng*. Take 1 *shēng* per dose warm, three doses per day.

- For palpitations in the heart, add 1.5 *liǎng* of guìzhī.
- For an exuberance of surging Qì, add 1.5 *liǎng* of wǔwèizǐ.
- For distressing dizziness in the head, add 1.5 *liǎng* of báizhú.
- For dry retching, remove the dàzǎo and add 1.5 *liǎng* of shēngjiāng instead.
- For center fullness, remove the dàzǎo.
- For a feeling in the heart like hunger, restore the use of dàzǎo.
- For cough with countercurrent movement and miserable headache, add 1.5 *liǎng* of xìxīn.
- For cold in the four limbs and difficult urination, add 1 piece of fùzǐ, blast-fried.

大補肝湯

治肝氣虛，其人恐懼不安，氣自少腹上衝咽，呃聲不止，頭目苦眩，不能坐起，汗出，心悸，乾嘔不能食，脈弱而結者方:

桂枝	
乾薑	
五味子	各三兩
旋覆花	
代赭石（一方作牡丹皮，當從）	
竹葉	各一兩
大棗（去核，一方作薯蕷，；當從）	十二枚

上七味，以水一斗，煮取四升，溫服一升，日三夜一服。

Dà Bǔ Gān Tāng
(Major Liver-Supplementing Decoction)

A formula to treat liver Qì vacuity, which causes the person to experience fear and being startled and not at ease, Qì surging up from the lower abdomen into the throat, incessant hiccup with noise, miserable dizzy head and vision, inability to sit or stand up, sweating, heart palpitations, dry retching and inability to eat, and a weak and bound pulse:

guìzhī	
gānjiāng	
wǔwèizǐ	3 *liǎng* each
xuánfùhuā	
dàizhěshí (an alternate [version of this] formula calls for mǔdānpí instead. Follow that!)	
zhúyè	1 *liǎng* each
dàzǎo (pitted. An alternate [version of this formula] calls for shǔyù instead. Follow that!)	12 pieces

Decoct the seven ingredients above in 1 *dǒu* of water until reduced to 4 *shēng*. Take 1 *shēng* per dose warm, three times a day and once at night.

1.3

Differentiating Patterns of Heart Disease: Essay and Formulas

辨心臟病證文並方

心虛則悲不已，心實則笑不休。

心病者，心胸內痛，脅下支滿，膺背肩胛間痛，兩臂內痛。虛則胸腹脅下與腰相引而痛。取其經手少陰、太陽，及舌下血者。其變，刺郗中血者。

邪在心，則病心中痛，善悲，時眩仆，視有餘不足而調之。經云：諸邪在心者，皆心胞代受，故證如是。

Vacuity in the heart results in never-ending grief. Repletion in the heart results in unstoppable laughter.

Illness of the heart invariably manifests with pain inside the heart and chest, propping fullness below the rib-sides, pain in the area of breasts, back, and shoulder blades, and pain inside both arms. Vacuity results in mutual pulling and pain in the chest, abdomen, below the rib-sides, and the lumbar area. Choose its channels, the Hand Shàoyīn and Tàiyáng, and draw blood below the tongue. For its pathological transformations, pierce the center of the cleft (i.e. Yīnxī, HT-6), drawing blood.

The presence of evil in the heart results in suffering from pain in the center of the heart, a tendency to grief, and periodic dizziness and falling over. See whether there is excess or insufficiency, and attune it accordingly. The Classic states: For the various sorts of evil in the heart, the pericardium always contracts them instead. Thus, the patterns are like this.

Translator's Note

This essay combines quotations from various *Nèijīng* chapters:

Língshū 《靈樞》 *8:*
心氣虛則悲；實則笑不休。

Vacuity in the heart results in grief. Repletion results in unstoppable laughter.

Sùwèn 《素問》 *22:*
心病者，胸中痛，脅支滿，脅下痛，膺背肩甲間痛，

兩臂內痛，虛則胸腹大，脅下與腰相引而痛，取其經，少陰太陽，舌下血者。其變病，刺郗中血者。

Illness of the heart invariably manifests with pain in the center of the chest, propping fullness in the rib-sides, pain below the rib-sides, pain in the area of breasts, back, and shoulder blades, and pain inside both arms. Vacuity results in an enlarged chest and abdomen, mutual pulling and pain in the region below the rib-sides and the lumbar area. Choose its channel, the Shàoyīn and the Tàiyáng, and draw blood below the tongue. For its pathological transformations, pierce the center of the cleft (i.e. Yīnxī, HT-6), drawing blood.

Língshū 《靈樞》 20:
邪在心，則病心痛喜悲，時眩仆，視有餘不足而調之其輸也。

The presence of evil in the heart results in suffering from pain in the heart, a tendency to grief, and periodic dizziness and falling over. See whether there is excess or insufficiency, and attune it accordingly at its shū *transport points.*

Língshū 《靈樞》 71:
黃帝曰：手少陰之脈，獨無俞，何也？歧伯曰：少陰，心脈也。心者，五藏六府之大主也，精神之所舍也，其藏堅固，邪弗能容也。容之則心傷，心傷則神去，神去則死矣。故諸邪之在於心者，皆在於心之包絡。

The Yellow Emperor asked: Why is it that the Hand Shàoyīn Vessel alone does not have holes? Qí Bó answered: Shàoyīn is the heart vessel. The heart is the supreme ruler of the five zàng *and six* fǔ *organs, and the residence of the* jīngshén*. Its* zàng *organ is solid and secure and evil cannot be contained in it. When it contains evil, the heart sustains* *damage, and when the heart is damaged, the Shén leaves, and when the Shén leaves, the result is death! For this reason, the presence of the various evils in the heart always means that they are present in the pericardium network vessels of the heart.*

陶云：心德在耎。故經云：以鹹補之，
苦瀉之。心苦緩，急食酸以收之。

Táo [Hóngjǐng] states: The special power of the heart lies in softness. Therefore the Classic says to use the salty flavor to supplement it and the bitter flavor to drain it. When the heart suffers from slackening, urgently consume sour substances to contract it.

Translator's Note

This quotation of the "Classic" refers to *Sùwèn* 《素問》 22:

心欲耎，急食鹹以耎之，用鹹補之，甘瀉之。

The heart desires softness. Quickly consume salty substances to soften it. Use the salty flavor to supplement it and the sweet flavor to drain it.

小瀉心湯

治心中卒急痛，脅下支滿，氣逆攻膺背肩胛間，不可飲食，食之反篤者方：

龍膽草	
梔子（打）	各三兩
戎鹽（如杏子大，燒赤）	三枚

上三味，以酢三升，煮取一升，頓服。少頃，得吐瘥。

Xiǎo Xiè Xīn Tāng
(Minor Heart-Draining Decoction)

A formula to treat sudden tense pain in the center of the heart, propping fullness below the rib-sides, Qì moving countercurrent to attack the area between the breast, back, and shoulder blades, and inability to eat and drink, with the condition intensifying contrary [to expectations] after eating:

lóngdǎncǎo	
zhīzǐ (broken into pieces)	3 *liǎng* each
róngyán (the size of apricot seeds, roasted until red)	3 pieces

Decoct the three ingredients above in 3 *shēng* of vinegar until reduced to 1 *shēng*. Quaff in a single dose. After a few moments, achieving vomiting means recovery.

Translator's Note

There are two versions of Xiǎo Xiè Xīn Tāng (Minor Heart-Draining Decoction) found in this text, which are identical in name but different in content. They furthermore differ from any heart-draining formulas in the *Shānghánlùn* 《傷寒論》 and *Jīnguì yàolüe* 《金匱要略》.

大瀉心湯

治暴得心腹痛，痛如刀刺，欲吐不吐，欲下不下，心中懊憹，脅背胸支滿迫急不可奈者方：

龍膽草	
梔子（擣）	各三兩
苦參	
升麻	各二兩
豉	半升
戎鹽（如大杏子大）	三枚

上六味，以酢六升，先煮上五味，得三升許，去滓。內戎鹽，稍煮待消已，取二升，服一升。當大吐，吐已必自瀉下，即瘥。（一方無苦參，有通草二兩，當從。）

Dà Xiè Xīn Tāng
(Major Heart-Draining Decoction)

A formula to treat fulminant contraction of heart and abdominal pain, with pain as if being stabbed with a knife, being on the verge of vomiting without actually doing so, being on the verge of downward elimination without actually doing so, anguish in the heart, and propping fullness in the rib-sides, back, and chest with such distressing urgency as to be unbearable:

lóngdǎncǎo	
zhīzǐ (pestled)	3 *liǎng* each
kǔshēn	
shēngmá	2 *liǎng* each
dàndòuchǐ	0.5 *shēng*
róngyán (the size of big apricot seeds)	3 pieces

Of the six ingredients above, first decoct the first five in 6 *shēng* of vinegar until reduced to about 3 *shēng* and remove the dregs. Add the róngyán and boil [the decoction] a bit more until [the salt] is dissolved and [the decoction] is reduced to 2 *shēng*. Take 1 *shēng* per dose. There must be great vomiting, and when the vomiting is done, there must be spontaneous diarrhea below. This means recovery. (An alternate [version of this] formula does not have kǔshēn but has 2 *liǎng* of tōngcǎo instead. Follow that!)

小補心湯

治胸痹不得臥，心痛徹背，背痛徹心者方：

栝蔞（擣）	一枚
薤白	八兩
半夏（洗去滑）	半斤

上三味，以白截漿一斗，煮取四升，溫服一升，日再服。（一方有杏仁，無半夏，熬）

Xiǎo Bǔ Xīn Tāng
(Minor Heart-Supplementing Decoction)

A formula to treat chest *bì* Impediment with inability to lie down, with heart pain that is penetrating through to the back, and back pain that is penetrating through to the heart:

guālóu (pestled)	1 piece
xièbái	8 *liǎng*
bànxià (washed until no longer slippery)	0.5 *jīn*

Decoct the three ingredients above in 1 *dǒu* of fermented rice drink until reduced to 4 *shēng*. Take 1 *shēng* per dose warm, two doses per day. (An alternate [version of this] formula has xìngrén, slowly toasted, instead of bànxià.)

Translator's Note

This formula is identical in ingredients and indications with the formula for Guālóu Xièbái Bànxià Tāng in the *Shānghánlùn* 《傷寒論》. The only difference is that that version calls for simmering the herbs in 1 *dǒu* of white rice wine, instead of the fermented rice drink mentioned here.

大補心湯

治胸痹，心中痞滿，氣結在胸，時從脅下逆搶心，心痛無奈方：

栝蔞（擣）	一枚
薤白	八兩
半夏（洗去滑）	半升
枳實（熬）	二兩
厚朴（炙）	二兩
桂枝	一兩

上六味，以白截漿一斗，煮取四升，每服二升，日再。（一方有杏仁半升，熬，無半夏，當從）

Dà Bǔ Xīn Tāng
(Major Heart-Supplementing Decoction)

A formula to treat chest *bì* Impediment, *pǐ* Glomus fullness in the center of the heart, Qì binding in the chest and periodically moving countercurrent from below the rib-sides to knock against the heart, and heart pain that is unbearable:

guālóu (pestled)	1 piece
xièbái	8 *liǎng*
bànxià (washed until no longer slippery)	0.5 *shēng*
zhǐshí (slowly toasted)	2 *liǎng*
hòupò (mix-fried)	2 *liǎng*
guìzhī	1 *liǎng*

Decoct the six ingredients above in 1 *dǒu* of fermented rice drink until reduced to 4 *shēng*. Take 2 *shēng* per dose, two doses per day. (An alternate [version of this] formula has 0.5 *shēng* of xìngrén, slowly toasted, and no bànxià. Follow that!)

心胞氣實者，受外邪之動也。則胸脅支滿，心中澹澹大動，面赤，目黃，善笑不休。虛則血氣少，善悲，久不已，發癲仆。

When the pericardium Qì is replete, this means that it has contracted the stirring of external evil. This results in propping fullness in the chest and rib-sides, turbulence in the heart and great stirring, a red face, yellow eyes, and a tendency to laugh without stopping. When it is vacuous, the result is shortage of blood and Qì and a tendency to grief, which are chronic and never-ending, and episodes of convulsions and falling.

小瀉心湯

治胸腹支滿，心中跳動不安者方：

黃連	
黃芩	
大黃	各三兩

上三味，以麻沸湯三升，漬一食頃，絞去滓，頓服。

Xiǎo Xiè Xīn Tāng
(Minor Heart-Draining Decoction)

A formula to treat propping fullness in the chest and abdomen and twitching and restlessness in the heart:

huánglián	
huángqín	
dàhuáng	3 *liǎng* each

Soak the three ingredients above in 3 *shēng* of boiling hot water for the length of time it takes to eat a meal. Wring out and remove the dregs. Quaff in a single dose.

Translator's Note

This formula for Xiǎo Xìe Xīn Tāng is identical in composition and similar in indications to a formula called Sān Huáng Tāng (Three Yellows Decoction) found in the *Zhōngcángjīng* 《中藏經》 (Classic stored in the center), a medieval text of unknown date or authorship.

大瀉心湯

治心中怔忡不安，胸膺痞懣，口中苦，舌上生瘡，面赤如新妝，或吐血、衄血、下血者方：

黃連	
黃芩	
芍藥	各三兩
乾薑（炮）	
甘草（炙）	
大黃	各三兩

上六味，以水五升，煮取二升，溫分再服，日二。

Dà Xiè Xīn Tāng
(Major Heart-Draining Decoction)

A formula to treat fearful throbbing and restlessness in the heart, *pǐ* Glomus fullness in the anterior chest, bitterness in the mouth, the formation of sores on top of the tongue, a red face like freshly applied make-up, and possibly vomiting blood or nosebleed or bleeding below:

huánglián	
huángqín	
sháoyào	3 *liǎng* each
gānjiāng (blast-fried)	
gāncǎo (mix-fried)	
dàhuáng	3 *liǎng* each

Decoct the six ingredients above in 5 *shēng* of water until reduced to 2 *shēng*. Take warm, divided in half, two doses a day.

小補心湯

治血氣虛少，心中動悸，時悲泣，煩躁，汗出，氣噫，脈結者方：

代赭石（燒赤，入酢漿中淬三次，打。 一方作牡丹皮，當從）	
旋覆花	
竹葉	各二兩
豉（一方作山萸肉，當從）	一兩

上方四味，以水八升，煮取三升，溫服一升，日三服。

- 怔忡不安者，加代赭石，為四兩半；
- 煩熱汗出者，去豉，加竹葉至四兩半，身熱還用豉；
- 心中窒痛者，加豉至四兩半；
- 氣苦少者，加甘草三兩；
- 心下痞滿者，去豉，加人參一兩半；
- 胸中冷而多唾者，加乾薑一兩半；
- 咽中介介塞者，加旋覆花至四兩半。

Xiǎo Bǔ Xīn Tāng
(Minor Heart-Supplementing Decoction)

A formula to treat blood and Qì vacuity and lack, stirring and palpitation in the heart, periodic grief and weeping, vexation and agitation, sweating, belching, and a bound pulse:

dàizhěshí (roasted until red, quenched three times in fermented rice drink, and broken into pieces. An alternate [version of this] formula calls for mǔdānpí instead. Follow that!)	
xuánfùhuā	
zhúyè	2 *liǎng* each
dàndòuchǐ (An alternate [version of this] formula calls for shānyúròu instead. Follow that!)	1 *liǎng*

Decoct the four ingredients in the formula above in 8 *shēng* of water until reduced to 3 *shēng* and take 1 *shēng* per dose warm, three doses a day.

- For fearful throbbing and restlessness, increase dàizhěshí to a total of 4.5 *liǎng*.
- For vexation heat and sweating, remove the dàndòuchǐ and increase the zhúyè to 4.5 *liǎng*. If there is generalized heat, keep the dàndòuchǐ.
- For blockage and pain in the heart, increase the dàndòuchǐ to 4.5 *liǎng*.
- For miserable scantness of Qì, add 3 *liǎng* of gāncǎo.
- For *pǐ* Glomus fullness below the heart, remove the dàndòuchǐ and add 1.5 *liǎng* of rénshēn.
- For cold in the chest with a lot of spittle, add 1.5 *liǎng* of gānjiāng.

- For stubborn obstruction in the throat, increase the xuánfùhuā to 4.5 *liǎng*.

Translator's Note

An alternate version of this text has 「心下痞满」 ("*pǐ* Glomus fullness below the heart") instead of "blockage and pain in the center of the heart" for the third modification of this formula. This is most likely a typographical error since that symptom is the indication for another modification further down.

大補心湯

治心中虛煩，懊怔不發，怔忡如車馬驚，飲食無味，乾嘔，氣噫，時或多唾，其人脈結而微者方：

代赭石（燒赤，入酢漿中淬三次，打。一方作牡丹皮，當從）	
旋覆花	
竹葉	各三兩
豉（一方作山萸肉，當從）	
人參	
甘草（炙）	
乾薑	各一兩

上方七味，以水一斗，煮取四升，溫服一升，日三夜一服。

Dà Bǔ Xīn Tāng
(Major Heart-Supplementing Decoction)

A formula to treat vacuity vexation in the heart, anguish and dread that fail to effuse, fearful throbbing like a panicking chariot horse, no appetite for food and drink, dry retching, belching, occasionally a lot of spittle, and a pulse that is bound and faint in such a person:

dàizhěshí (roasted until red, quenched three times in fermented rice drink, and broken into pieces. An alternate [version of this] formula calls for mǔdānpí instead. Follow that!)	
xuánfùhuā	
zhúyè	3 *liǎng* each
dàndòuchǐ (An alternate [version of this] formula calls for shānyúròu instead. Follow that!)	
rénshēn	
gāncǎo (mix-fried)	
gānjiāng	1 *liǎng* each

Decoct the seven ingredients of the formula above in 1 *dǒu* of water until reduced to 4 *shēng*. Take warm, 1 *shēng* per dose, three doses a day and one at night.

1.4

Differentiating Patterns of Spleen Disease: Essay and Formulas

辨脾臟病證文並方

脾實則腹滿，飧泄；虛則四肢不用，五臟不安。

脾病者，必腹滿腸鳴，溏瀉，食不化。虛則身重，若飢，肉痛，足痿不收，行善瘈，腳下痛。

邪在脾，則肌肉痛。陽氣不足，則寒中，腸鳴，腹痛；陰氣不足，則善飢。皆調其三里。

Repletion in the spleen results in abdominal fullness and dinner-time diarrhea. Vacuity results in inability to use the four limbs and restlessness in the five *zàng* organs.

Illness of the spleen invariably manifests in abdominal fullness with rumbling intestines, sloppy diarrhea, and failure to transform food. Vacuity results in heaviness of the body, a sensation like starving, pain in the flesh, wilting and inability to contract [the muscles of] the lower legs, a tendency to spasms when walking, and pain below the feet.

The presence of evil in the spleen results in pain in the flesh and skin. Insufficiency of Yáng Qì results in cold in the center, rumbling intestines, and abdominal pain. Insufficiency of Yīn Qì results in a tendency to feel starved. In all cases, attune the patient's Sānlǐ points (LI-10 and ST-36).

Translator's Note

This essay combines quotations from various *Nèijīng* chapters:

Língshū 《靈樞》 *8:*
脾氣虛則四肢不用，五藏不安；實則
腹脹，經溲不利。

Vacuity of spleen Qì results in inability to use the four limbs and restlessness in the five zàng *organs. Repletion results in abdominal distention and inhibited menstruation and urination.*

Sùwèn 《素問》 22:

脾病者，身重善肌肉痿，足不收行，善瘛，腳下痛，虛則腹滿腸鳴，飧泄食不化，取其經，太陰、陽明、少陰血者。

Illness of the spleen invariably manifests with generalized heaviness, a tendency to wilting in the flesh, failure to contract [the muscles of] the lower legs to walk, a tendency to convulsions, and pain below the feet. Vacuity results in abdominal fullness and rumbling intestines, dinner-time diarrhea, and failure to transform food. Choose its channels, tàiyīn and yángmíng and shàoyīn, and draw blood.

Língshū 《靈樞》 20:

邪在脾胃，則病肌肉痛。陽氣有餘，陰氣不足，則熱中善饑；陽氣不足，陰氣有餘，則寒中腸鳴腹痛；陰陽俱有餘，若俱不足，則有寒有熱。皆調於三里。

The presence of evil in the spleen and stomach results in suffering from pain in the flesh and skin. In cases with excess of Yáng Qì and insufficiency of Yīn Qì, the result is heat in the center and a tendence to feel starved. In cases with an insufficiency of Yáng Qì and excess of Yīn Qì, the result is cold in the center, rumbling intestines, and abdominal pain. When there is an excess of both Yīn and Yáng, or an insufficiency of both, then there is cold and there is heat. In all cases, attune [the patient's Qì] at the Sānlǐ points (LI-10 and ST-36).

陶云：脾德在緩。故經云：以甘補之，
辛瀉之。脾苦濕，急食苦以燥之。

Táo [Hóngjǐng] states: The special power of the spleen lies in slackening. Therefore the Classic says to use the sweet flavor to supplement it and the acrid flavor to drain it. When the spleen suffers from dampness, urgently consume bitter substances to dry it out.

Translator's Note

This quotation from the "Classic" refers to *Sùwèn* 《素問》 22:

脾欲緩，急食甘以緩之，用苦瀉之，甘補之。

The spleen desires slackness. Urgently consume sweet substances to slacken it, and use bitter substances to drain it and sweet substances to supplement it.

小瀉脾湯

治脾氣實，下利清穀，裡寒外熱，腹冷，脈微者方：

附子（炮）	一枚
乾薑	
甘草（炙）	各三兩

上三味，以水三升，煮取一升，頓服。

Xiǎo Xiè Pí Tāng
(Minor Spleen-Draining Decoction)

A formula to treat spleen Qì repletion, with clear-grain diarrhea, interior cold and heat on the outside, coolness in the abdomen, and a faint pulse:

fùzǐ (blast-fried)	1 piece
gānjiāng	
gāncǎo (mix-fried)	3 *liǎng* each

Decoct the three ingredients above in 3 *shēng* of water until reduced to 1 *shēng*. Quaff in a single dose.

Translator's Note

This formula is identical in ingredients and similar in indications to Tōng Mài Sì Nì Tāng 通脈四逆湯 (Vessel-Freeing Fourfold Counter-current Decoction) from the *Shānghánlùn* 《傷寒論》. Even though it is here indicated as a treatment for spleen Qì repletion, and thus called "Spleen-Draining Decoction," its key symptoms are all signs of spleen Qì vacuity cold and it is actually a drastic intervention to supplement the spleen's Yáng Qì.

大瀉脾湯

治腹中脹滿，乾嘔不能食，欲利不得，或下利不止者方：

附子（炮）	一枚
乾薑	三兩
黃芩	
大黃	
枳實	
甘草（炙）	各一兩

上方六味，以水五升，煮取二升，溫分再服，日二。

Dà Xiè Pí Tāng
(Major Spleen-Draining Decoction)

A formula to treat distention and fullness in the abdomen, dry retching and inability to eat, wanting to have diarrhea but not being able to, or diarrhea that is unstoppable:

fùzǐ (blast-fried)	1 piece
gānjiāng	3 *liǎng*
huángqín	
dàhuáng	
zhǐshí	
gāncǎo (mix-fried)	1 *liǎng* each

Decoct the six ingredients of the formula above in 5 *shēng* of water until reduced to 2 *shēng*. Take warm, divided in half, two doses a day.

Translator's Note

The manuscript version of this formula originally contained gāncǎo, which was later replaced with sháoyào. The remaining five ingredients are identical to the edition memorized by Zhāng Dàcháng. The authors of *Dūnhuáng gǔyījí kǎoshì* (Philological Study of the Dunhuang Medical Records) point out that in accordance with the pattern of the rest of this text, all five of the major *zàng* organ-draining decoctions are composed of six medicinal ingredients, of which five are identical in all of them, namely: gān/shēngjiāng, sháoyào, dàhuáng, huángqín, and gāncǎo. In each formula, there is only one ingredient that is different, which is derived from the formula for the related "Minor *zàng* Organ-Draining Decoction." Following this rule, the formula above should contain these five shared ingredients but should not include zhǐshí, which is the defining medicinal for the liver-draining decoctions.

小補脾湯

治飲食不化，時自吐利，吐利已，心中苦飢，或心下痞滿，脈微無力，身重，足痿，善轉筋者方：

人參	
甘草（炙）	
乾薑	各三兩
白朮	一兩

上四味，以水八升，煮取三升，分三服，日三。

- 苦臍上築動者，去朮，加桂四兩；
- 吐多者，去朮，加生薑三兩；
- 下多者，仍用朮；
- 心中悸者，加茯苓一分［兩］；
- 渴欲飲者，加朮至四兩半；
- 腹中滿者，去朮，加附子，一枚，炮；
- 腹中痛者，加人參一分；
- 寒者，加乾薑一分。

Xiǎo Bǔ Pí Tāng
(Minor Spleen-Supplementing Decoction)

A formula to treat failure to transform food and drink, periodic spontaneous vomiting and diarrhea, miserable hunger in the heart when the vomiting and diarrhea are finished, possibly *pǐ* Glomus fullness below the heart, a pulse that is faint and lacking strength, heaviness of the body, wilting in the lower legs, and a tendency to twisting sinews:

rénshēn	
gāncǎo (mix-fried)	
gānjiāng	3 *liǎng* each
báizhú	1 *liǎng*

Decoct the four ingredients above in 8 *shēng* of water until reduced to 3 *shēng*. Divide into three doses and take three times a day.

- For miserable pounding above the navel, remove the báizhú and add 4 *liǎng* of guìzhī instead.
- For an increase in vomiting, remove the báizhú and add 3 *liǎng* of shēngjiāng instead.
- For an increase in downward movement, keep the báizhú [in the formula].
- For palpitations in the heart, add 1 *fēn* of fúlíng.
- For thirst with desire to drink, increase the báizhú to 4.5 *liǎng*.
- For fullness in the abdomen, remove the báizhú and add 1 piece of fùzǐ, blast-fried, instead.
- For pain in the abdomen, add 1 *fēn* of rénshēn.
- For cold, add 1 *fēn* of gānjiāng.

Translator's Note

The present formula is clearly related to Lǐ Zhōng Wán (Center-Patterning Pill) in the *Shānghánlùn*, where it is listed in the chapter on "Sudden Turmoil." The two formulas are identical in terms of the ingredients, the preparation instructions as a decoction, and the modifications. The major difference is that the *Shānghánlùn* version calls for 3 *liǎng* each of all the ingredients. In addition, those instructions call for these to be pounded and sifted, processed into honey pills, and taken in hot liquid numerous times during the day and night, with the dosage to be increased until there is a sensation of heat in the abdomen. the text then goes on to state that the pill preparation is not as good as the decoction, the instructions for which are literally identical to the ones given for Xiǎo Bǔ Pí Tāng in the present text.

In terms of the measurements for the modifications, according to the *Běncǎojīng jízhù*, 4 *fēn* constitute 1 *liǎng*. This contrasts, however, with the amounts given for Lǐ Zhōng Wán in the *Shānghánlùn*, where palpitations in the heart are treated with the addition of 2 *liǎng* of fúlíng. The final two modifications, for pain in the abdomen and for cold, are missing there, while the other modifications are almost literally identical in both texts. Lastly the *Shānghánlùn* version says to "wait for the duration of a meal after taking the decoction and then drink down about 1 *shēng* of hot gruel to induce mild warmth and stay covered up with clothes and blankets."

The striking overlap between these two texts shows that they were most likely based on a shared source that has since been lost.

大補脾湯

治脾氣大疲，飲食不化，嘔吐下利，其人枯瘦如柴，立不可動轉，口中苦乾渴，汗出，氣急，脈微而時結者方：

人參	
甘草（炙）	各三兩
乾薑	三兩
朮	
麥門冬	
五味子	
旋覆花（一方作牡丹皮，當從）	各一兩

上七味，以水一斗，煮取四升，溫分四服，日三夜一服。

Dà Bǔ Pí Tāng
(Major Spleen-Supplementing Decoction)

A formula to treat major exhaustion of spleen Qì, failure to transform food and drink, retching, vomiting, and diarrhea, bone-dry emaciation of the patient until they look like sticks and bones, inability to turn sides when standing, miserable dryness and thirst in the mouth, sweating, urgent breathing, and a pulse that is faint and periodically bound:

rénshēn	
gāncǎo (mix-fried)	3 *liǎng* each
gānjiāng	3 *liǎng*
báizhú	
màiméndōng	
wǔwèizǐ	
xuánfùhuā (an alternate [version of this] formula calls for mǔdānpí instead. Follow that!)	1 *liǎng* each

Decoct the seven ingredients above in 1 *dǒu* of water until reduced to 4 *shēng*. Take it warm, divided into four doses, three times a day and once at night.

1.5

Differentiating Patterns of Lung Disease: Essay and Formulas

辨肺臟病證候文並方

肺虛則鼻息不利；實則喘咳，憑胸仰息。

肺病者，必咳喘逆氣，肩息，背痛，汗出憎風。虛則胸中痛，少氣，不能報息，耳聾，咽乾。

邪在肺，則皮膚痛，發寒熱，上氣喘，汗出，咳動肩背。取之膺中外腧，背第三椎旁，以手按之快然，乃刺之，取缺盆以越之。

Vacuity in the lung results in inhibited breathing through the nose. Repletion results in panting and cough and in fullness in the chest and breathing [only] with the head tilted up.

Illness of the lung invariably manifests with cough and panting with countercurrent movement of Qì, breathing with raised shoulders, back pain, sweating, and an abhorrence of wind. Vacuity results in pain in the chest, scantness of breath, inability to breathe in and out continuously, deafness, and dry throat.

The presence of evil in the lung results in pain in the skin, effusion of cold and heat, Qì ascent and panting, sweating, and cough that is [so intense as to] stir up the shoulders and back. Capture it at the outer *shù* Transport points in the chest, and on the back next to the third vertebra. Needle it when pressing down [on the point] with your hand elicits a comfortable feeling. Capture [it at] Quēpén (ST-12) in order to scatter it.

Translator's Note

This essay combines quotations from various *Nèijīng* chapters:

Língshū 《靈樞》 8:
肺藏氣，氣舍魄，肺氣虛則鼻塞不利少氣；
實則喘喝，胸盈仰息。

The lung stores the Qì, and Qì houses the pò *souls. Vacuity in the lung results in nasal congestion and scantness of breath. Repletion results in panting and coughing, fullness in the chest, and breathing [only] with the head tilted up.*

Sùwèn 《素問》 22:

肺病者，喘咳逆氣，肩背痛，汗出，尻陰股膝髀腨足皆痛，虛則少氣不能報息，耳聾嗌乾。取其經，太陰、足太陽之外厥陰內血者。

Illness of the lung invariably manifests with panting and cough with countercurrent movement of Qì, pain in the shoulders and back, sweating, and pain in the end of the spine, genitals, thighs, knees, thigh bones, shins, calves, and feet, all of these places. Vacuity results in scantness of breath and inability to breathe in and out continuously, deafness, choking and dryness [in the throat]. Choose its channels, Tàiyīn and the outside of Foot Tàiyáng and inside of Juèyīn and draw blood.

Língshū 《靈樞》 20:

邪在肺，則病皮膚痛，寒熱，上氣喘，汗出，咳動肩背。取之膺中外俞，背三節五藏之傍，以手疾按之，快然，乃刺之，取之缺盆中以越之。

The presence of evil in the lung results in pain in the skin, cold and heat, Qì ascent and panting, sweating, and cough that is [so intense as to] stir up the shoulders and back. Capture it at the outer shù *transport points in the chest, and on the side of the third vertebra on the back. Needle it when pressing down urgently [on the point] with your hand elicits a comfortable feeling. Capture it in the center of Quēpén in order to scatter it.*

According to commentary tradition, the "outer *shù* transport points in the chest" is a reference to the two points Yúnmén 雲門 (LU-2) and Zhōngfǔ 中府 (LU-1).

陶云：肺德在收。故經云：以酸補之，鹹瀉之。肺苦氣上逆，食辛以散之，開腠理以通氣也。

Táo [Hóngjǐng] states: The special power of the lung lies in drawing inward. Therefore the Classic says to use the sour flavor to supplement it and to use the salty flavor to drain it. If the lung suffers from Qì ascending counter-current, consume acrid substances to disperse it and open the *còulǐ* Interstices, in order to restore the through-flow of Qì.

Translator's Note

This quotation from the "Classic" refers to *Sùwèn* 《素問》 22:

肺欲收，急食酸以收之。用酸補之，辛瀉之。

The lung desires drawing inward. Urgently consume sour substances to draw it inward. Use sour substances to supplement it, and acrid substances to drain it.

The textual discrepancy between these two sources in terms of draining the lung by means of salty versus sour substances is interesting for clinical practitioners. Unfortunately, it is impossible at this point to determine which version is closer to the original and therefore the correct one. This is not an instance where different editions of the *Sùwèn* differ from each other. Moreover, other quotations of this famous passage, such as Sūn Sīmiǎo's version in the *Bèijí qiānjīn yàofāng* volume on dietetics, follow the standard *Sùwèn* version and use acrid to drain it. My personal guess is therefore that this may be an error in the present text. Nevertheless, it is significant that the original compiler of our text made this substitution or error, if that is what it is, and that the numerous copiers afterwards through the centuries did not take it upon themselves to correct it, because they must surely have been familiar with the standard version of this passage from the *Sùwèn*.

小瀉肺湯

治咳喘上氣，胸中迫滿，不可臥者方：

葶藶子（熬黑，擣如泥）	
大黃	
芍藥	各三兩

上三味，以水三升，煮取二升，溫分再服，喘定止後服。

Xiǎo Xiè Fèi Tāng
(Minor Lung-Draining Decoction)

A formula to treat cough with panting, ascent of Qì, and distressing fullness in the chest, [so bad as to] prevent the patient from lying down:

tínglìzǐ (slowly toasted until black, pestled until it is like mud)	
dàhuáng	
sháoyào	3 *liǎng* each

Decoct the three ingredients above in 3 *shēng* of water until reduced to 2 *shēng*. Take warm, divided in half, in two doses. When the panting settles down, stop subsequent doses.

大瀉肺湯

治胸中有痰涎，喘不得臥，大小便悶，身面腫迫滿，欲得氣利者方：

葶藶子（熬）	
大黃	
芍藥	各二兩
甘草（炙）	
黃芩	
乾薑	各一兩

上六味，以水五升，煮取二升，溫分再服，日二服。

Dà Xiè Fèi Tāng
(Major Lung-Draining Decoction)

A formula to treat drastic drool in the chest, panting [so bad as to] prevent the patient from lying down, confined defecation and urination, swelling and distressing fullness in the whole body and face, and desire to achieve an uninhibited movement of Qì:

tínglìzǐ (slowly toasted)	
dàhuáng	
sháoyào	2 *liǎng* each
gāncǎo (mix-fried)	
huángqín	
gānjiāng	1 *liǎng* each

Decoct the six ingredients above in 5 *shēng* of water until reduced to 2 *shēng*. Take warm, divided in half, in two doses a day.

小補肺湯

治汗出口渴，少氣不足息，胸中痛，脈虛者方：

麥門冬	
五味子	
旋覆花（一方作牡丹皮，當從）	各三兩
細辛	一兩

上四味，以水八升，煮取三升，每服一升，日三服。

- 若胸中煩熱者，去細辛，加海蛤一兩；
- 若悶痛者，加細辛一兩；
- 咳疾不出，脈結者，倍旋覆花為六兩；
- 若眩冒者，去細辛，加澤瀉一兩；
- 咳而吐血者，倍麥門冬為六兩；
- 若煩渴者，去細辛，加粳米半升；
- 涎多者，仍用細辛，加半夏半升，洗。

Xiǎo Bǔ Fèi Tāng
(Minor Lung-Supplementing Decoction)

A formula to treat sweating with thirst, scantness of breath and insufficient Qì for breathing, pain in the chest, and a vacuous pulse:

màiméndōng	
wǔwèizǐ	
xuánfùhuā (an [alternate version of this] formula calls for mǔdānpí. Follow that!)	3 *liǎng* each
xìxīn	1 *liǎng*

Decoct the four ingredients above in 8 *shēng* of water until reduced to 3 *shēng*. Take 1 *shēng* per dose, three doses a day.

- For vexing heat in the chest, remove the xìxīn and add 1 *liǎng* of hǎigé instead.
- For oppression with pain, add 1 *liǎng* of xìxīn.
- For cough that is urgent but nonproductive, with a bound pulse, double the amount of xuánfùhuā to 6 *liǎng*.
- For veiling dizziness, remove the xìxīn and add 1 *liǎng* of zéxiè.
- For cough with vomiting blood, double the amount of màiméndōng to 6 *liǎng*.
- For vexing thirst, remove the xìxīn and add 0.5 *shēng* of jīngmǐ.
- For increased drool, keep the xìxīn but add 0.5 *shēng* of bànxià, washed.

Translator's Note

I have followed the editors of the version of this text printed in the *Dūnhuáng gǔījí kǎoshì* in reading the character 分 (*fēn*) used here as the measurement for hǎigé, xìxīn, and zéxiè as a typographical error that should be replaced with 兩 *liǎng*. I have also followed that edition and corrected the doubled amount of xuánfùhuā and màiméndōng, from "add 2 *liǎng*" to "6 *liǎng*" since the unmodified formula calls for 3 *liǎng*.

大補肺湯

治煩熱汗出，少氣不足息，口乾，耳聾，脈虛而快者方：

麥門冬	
五味子	
旋覆花（一方作牡丹皮，當從）	各三兩
細辛	一兩
地黃	
竹葉	
甘草	各一兩

上七味，以水一斗，煮取四升，溫分四服，日三夜一服。

Dà Bǔ Fèi Tāng
(Major Lung-Supplementing Decoction)

A formula to treat vexing heat with sweating, scantness of breath and insufficient Qì for breathing, dry mouth, deafness, and a vacuous and fast pulse:

màiméndōng	
wǔwèizǐ	
xuánfùhuā (an [alternate version of this] formula calls for mǔdānpí instead. Follow that!)	3 *liǎng* each
xìxīn	1 *liǎng*
dìhuáng	
zhúyè	
gāncǎo	1 *liǎng* each

Decoct the seven ingredients above in 1 *dǒu* of water until reduced to 4 *shēng*. Take warm, divided into four doses, three times a day and once at night.

1.6

Differentiating Patterns of Kidney Disease: Essay and Formulas

辨腎臟病證文並方

腎氣虛則厥逆，實則腹滿，面色正黑，涇溲不利。

腎病者，必腹大脛腫，身重，嗜寢。虛則腰中痛，大腹小腹痛，尻陰、股、膝攣，胻足皆痛。

邪在腎，則骨痛，陰痹。陰痹者，按之不得。腹脹，腰痛，大便難，肩背項強痛，時眩仆，取之湧泉，昆侖，視有餘血者盡取之。

Vacuity of kidney Qì results in reversal counter-current flow. Repletion results in abdominal fullness, a pure black facial complexion, and inhibited urination.

Illness of the kidney invariably manifests with an enlarged abdomen and swelling in the shins, generalized heaviness, and a craving for sleep. Vacuity results in pain in the middle of the lumbar area, pain in the upper and lower abdomen, hypertonicity in the end of the spine, genitals, thighs, and knees, and pain in the calves and feet, all of these places.

The presence of evil in the kidney results in pain in the bones and Yīn *bì* Impediment—Yīn *bì* Impediment meaning that when you press on it, you cannot get it—abdominal distention, lumbar pain, difficult defecation, rigidity and pain in the shoulders, back, and neck, and periodic dizziness with falling. Capture it at Yǒngquán (KI-1) and Kūnlún (BL-60). If you observe that there is residual blood, [make sure] to completely capture it.

Translator's Note

This essay combines quotations from various *Nèijīng* chapters:

Língshū 《靈樞》 *8:*

腎藏精，精舍志，腎氣虛則厥；實則脹，五藏不安。

The kidney stores the jīng *Essence, and the* jīng *Essence houses the will. Vacuity of kidney Qì results in reversal. Repletion results in distention and in restlessness in the five* zàng *organs.*

The last two symptoms (pure black facial complexion and inhibited urination) appear to be an addition by the authors of the present text, or could have been part of the original shared source predating the *Língshū*.

Sùwèn 《素問》 22:

腎病者，腹大脛腫，喘咳，身重，寢汗出憎風。虛則胸中痛，大腹小腹痛，清厥，意不樂。取其經，少陰太陽血者。

Illness of the kidney invariably manifests with an enlarged abdomen and swelling in the shins, panting and cough, generalized heaviness, sweating during sleep, and abhorrence of wind. Vacuity results in pain in the middle of the chest, pain in the upper and lower abdomen, cold with reversal, and lack of joy in the yì *intention. Choose its channels, the Shàoyīn and Tàiyáng, and draw blood.*

Língshū 《靈樞》 20:

邪在腎，則病骨痛陰痺。陰痺者，按之而不得，腹脹腰痛，大便難，肩背頸項痛，時眩。取之湧泉、崑崙，視有血者盡取之。

The presence of evil in the kidney results in being ill with bone pain and Yīn bì *Impediment—Yīn* bì *Impediment meaning that when you press on it, you cannot get it—abdominal distention, lumbar pain, difficult defecation, pain in the shoulders, back, and neck, and periodic dizziness. Capture it at Yǒngquán (KI-1) and Kūnlún (BL-60). If you observe that there is blood, [make sure] to completely capture it.*

陶云：腎德在堅。故經云：以苦補之，甘瀉之。腎苦燥，急食鹹以潤之，至津液生也。

Táo [Hóngjǐng] states: The special power of the kidney lies in hardening. Therefore the Classic says to use the bitter flavor to supplement it and to use the sweet flavor to drain it. When the kidney suffers from dryness, urgently consume salty substances to moisten it and cause the generation of fluids.

Translator's Note

This quotation from the "Classic" refers to *Sùwèn* 《素問》 22:

腎苦燥，急食辛以潤之，開腠理，致津液，
通氣也。。。腎欲堅，急食苦以堅之 。用
苦補之，鹹瀉之。

> *If the kidney suffers from dryness, quickly consume acrid substances to moisten it, open the* còulǐ, *cause the fluids to arrive, and make the Qì flow through... The kidney desires hardness. Urgently consume bitter substances to harden it. use the bitter flavor to supplement it and use the salty flavor to drain it.*

While the textual similarities make it clear that the compilers of the *Nèijīng* and our present text relied on a common source, or perhaps even on two different sources that derived from yet another shared ancestor, the discrepancies are significant and fascinating, both for historians and for clinicians. At this point, it is impossible to determine which version was earlier and therefore the "correct" one, but perhaps that is even the wrong question to ask in the first place. I invite you instead to contemplate the significance of these differences since they are bound to enrich our clinical perspective.

小瀉腎湯

治小便赤少，少腹滿，時足脛腫者方：

茯苓	
甘草	
黃芩	各三兩

上三味，以水三升，煮取一升，頓服。

Xiǎo Xiè Shèn Tāng
(Minor Kidney-Draining Decoction)

A formula to treat red scanty urine, fullness in the lower abdomen, and periodic swelling in the lower legs:

fúlíng	
gāncǎo	
huángqín	3 *liǎng* each

Decoct the three ingredients above in 3 *shēng* of water until reduced to 1 *shēng*. Quaff in a single dose.

大瀉腎湯

治小便赤少，時溺血，少腹迫滿而痛，腰如折，耳鳴者方：

茯苓	
甘草	
大黃	
黃芩	各三兩
芍藥	
乾薑	各一兩

上方六味，以水五升，煮取二升，日二溫服。

Dà Xiè Shèn Tāng
(Major Kidney-Draining Decoction)

A formula to treat red and scanty urine, periodic blood in the urine, distressing fullness and pain the lower abdomen, a feeling as if the lumbar area were about to snap, and tinnitus:

fúlíng	
gāncǎo	
dàhuáng	
huángqín	3 *liǎng* each
sháoyào	
gānjiāng	1 *liǎng* each

Decoct the six ingredients from the formula above in 5 *shēng* of water until reduced to 2 *shēng*. Take in two doses a day, warm.

小補腎湯

治虛勞失精，腰痛，骨蒸羸瘦，脈快者方：

地黃	
竹葉	
甘草	各三兩
澤瀉	一兩

上四味，以水八升，煮取三升，日三服。

- 若小便血者，去澤瀉，加地榆一兩；
- 若大便見血者，去澤瀉，加伏龍肝如雞子大；
- 若苦遺精者，易生地黃為熟地黃；
- 若小便冷，莖中痛，倍澤瀉為二兩；
- 少腹苦迫急者，去澤瀉，加牡丹皮一兩；
- 小便不利者，仍用澤瀉；
- 心煩者，加竹葉；
- 腹中熱者，加梔子十四枚，打。

Xiǎo Bǔ Shèn Tāng
(Minor Kidney-Supplementing Decoction)

A formula to treat vacuity taxation with loss of *jīng* Essence, lumbar pain, bone steaming and marked emaciation, and a fast pulse:

dìhuáng	
zhúyè	
gāncǎo	3 *liǎng* each
zéxiè	1 *liǎng*

Decoct the four ingredients above in 8 *shēng* of water until reduced to 3 *shēng*. Take in three doses a day.

- For blood in the urine, remove the zéxiè and add 1 *liǎng* of dìyú instead.
- For blood visible in the stool, remove the zéxiè and add a piece of fúlónggān the size of a chicken egg.
- For suffering from seminal emission, replace the shēngdìhuáng with shúdìhuáng.
- For urine that is cold and pain in the penis, double the amount of zéxiè to 2 *liǎng*.
- For suffering from distressing tension in the lesser abdomen, remove the zéxiè and add 1 *liǎng* of mǔdānpí.
- For inhibited urination, still use the zéxiè.
- For heart vexation, add zhúyè.
- For heat in the center of the abdomen, add 15 pieces of zhīzǐ, broken up.

大補腎湯

治精氣虛少，腰痛，骨痿，不可行走，虛熱衝逆，頭目眩，小便不利，脈軟而快者方：

地黃	
竹葉	
甘草	各三兩
澤瀉	
桂枝	
乾薑	
五味子	各一兩

上七味，以長流水一斗，煮取四升，溫分四服，日三服夜一服。

Dà Bǔ Shèn Tāng
(Major Kidney-Supplementing Decoction)

A formula to treat shortage of *jīng* Essence and Qì, lumbar pain, bone wilting, inability to walk, vacuity heat with surging countercurrent flow, dizziness of the head and eyes, inhibited urination, and a soft and fast pulse:

dìhuáng	
zhúyè	
gāncǎo	3 *liǎng* each
zéxiè	
guìzhī	
gānjiāng	
wǔwèizǐ	1 *liǎng* each

Decoct the seven ingredients above in 1 *dǒu* of water from a long-flowing source until reduced to 4 *shēng*. Divide and take warm in four doses, three doses a day and one at night.

Translator's Note

This is the end of the first section of the text. This section has offered four formulas for each of the five *zàng* organs: a major and a minor formula each for draining and for supplementing. With the four additional major and minor draining and supplementing formulas for the heart, we thus arrive at a total of 24 formulas.

Section Two

Five Formulas to Address Drainage of the Five *Zàng* Organs

陶曰：又有瀉方五首，以救諸病誤治，致生變亂者也。

Táo [Hóngjǐng] states: Moreover, there are five "drain formulas." These are a means to rescue [patients] from all sorts of erroneous treatments of disease, to summon life and transform disorder.

瀉肝湯

救誤用吐法，其人神氣素虛，有痰澼發動嘔吐不止，驚煩不寧方：

枳實（熬）	
芍藥	
代赭石（燒，一方作牡丹皮，當從）	
旋覆花	
竹葉	各三兩

上方五味，以水七升，煮取三升，溫分再服。

Xiè Gān Tāng
(Liver Drain Decoction)

A formula to rescue cases of erroneous use of the vomiting method in patients with a constitutional vacuity of Shén Qì, causing the presence of urgent *pì* Afflux with stirring, retching, and vomiting that will not stop, and panic vexation that will not calm down:

zhǐshí (slowly toasted)	
sháoyào	
dàizhěshí (roasted, (an [alternate version of this] formula calls for mǔdānpí instead. Follow that!)	
xuánfùhuā	
zhúyè	3 *liǎng* each

Decoct the five ingredients from the formula above in 7 *shēng* of water until reduced to 3 *shēng*. Take warm, divided into two doses.

Translator's Note

I follow Wiseman's *Practical Dictionary of Chinese Medicine* in translating the character 澼 *pì* as "Afflux" (but add the Pīnyīn for readers unfamiliar with his terminology). In early medical literature, this can refer either to a pathological and painful accumulation of water, usually in the compound 腸澼 ("intestinal *pì* Afflux"), or to dysentery, as the painful manifestation of contracting damp heat or seasonal evils.

瀉心湯

救誤用清下，其人陽氣素實，外邪乘虛陷入，致心下痞滿，食不下，利反不止，雷鳴腹痛方：

黃連	
黃芩	
人參	
甘草（炙）	
乾薑（一方有大棗）	各三兩

上方五味，以水七升，煮取三升，溫分再服

Xiè Xīn Tāng
(Heart Drain Decoction)

A formula to rescue cases of erroneous use of the clearing and downward-moving method in patients with a constitutional repletion of Yáng Qì, where external evil has taken advantage of vacuity to invade, causing *pǐ* Glomus fullness below the heart, inability to move food down, and contrarian diarrhea that will not stop, rumbling [intestines] and abdominal pain:

huánglián	
huángqín	
rénshēn	
gāncǎo (mix-fried)	
gānjiāng (an [alternate version of this] formula calls for dàzǎo)	3 *liǎng* each

Decoct the five ingredients from the formula above in 7 *shēng* of water until reduced to 3 *shēng*. Take warm, divided into two doses.

瀉脾湯

救誤用冷寒，其人陰氣素實，衛氣不通，致腹中滯脹，反寒不已方：

附子（炮）	
乾薑	
麥冬	
五味子	
旋覆花（一方有細辛三兩）	各三兩

上方五味，以水七升，煮取三升，溫分再服。

Xiè Pí Tāng
(Spleen Drain Decoction)

A formula to rescue cases of erroneous use of the cooling and cold method in patients with a constitutional repletion of Yīn Qì, where their *wèi* Defense Qì fails to flow through, causing stagnation and distention in the abdomen and and contrarian cold that will not abate:

fùzǐ (blast-fried)	
gānjiāng	
màiméndōng	
wǔwèizǐ	
xuánfùhuā (an [alternate version of this] formula calls for 3 *liǎng* of xìxīn instead)	3 *liǎng* each

Decoct the five ingredients from the formula above in 7 *shēng* of water until reduced to 3 *shēng*. Take warm, divided into two doses.

瀉肺湯

救誤用火法，其人血素躁，致令神識迷妄如痴，吐血、衄血、胸中煩滿，氣結方：

葶藶子（熬黑，擣如泥）	
大黃	
生地黃	
竹葉	
甘草	各三兩

上五味，以水七升，煮取三升，溫分再服。

Xiè Fèi Tāng
(Lung Drain Decoction)

A formula to rescue cases of erroneous use of the fire method in patients with a constitutional dryness in the blood, causing mental confusion resembling feeblemindedness, vomiting of blood, nosebleed, vexing fullness in the chest, and Qì bind:

tínglìzǐ (slowly toasted until black, pounded into a mud-like consistency	
dàhuáng	
shēngdìhuáng	
zhúyè	
gāncǎo	3 *liǎng* each

Decoct the five ingredients above in 7 *shēng* of water until reduced to 3 *shēng*. Take warm, divided into two doses.

瀉腎湯

救誤用汗法，其人陽氣素虛，致令陰氣逆升，心中悸動不安，冒，汗出不止方：

茯苓	
甘草	
桂枝	
生薑	
五味子	各三兩

上方五味，以水七升，煮取三升，溫分再服。

Xiè Shèn Tāng
(Kidney Drain Decoction)

A formula to rescue cases of erroneous use of the sweating method in patients with a constitutional vacuity of Yáng Qì, causing the Yīn Qì to ascend counter-current, with palpitations, stirring, and restlessness in the heart, veiling, and sweating that will not stop:

fúlíng	
gāncǎo	
guìzhī	
shēngjiāng	
wǔwèizǐ	3 *liǎng* each

Decoct the five ingredients from the formula above in 7 *shēng* of water until reduced to 3 *shēng*. Take warm, divided into two doses.

Translator's Note

The five formulas above treat cases where medical therapies were applied incorrectly and, in combination with a constitutional imbalance, caused pathological changes in the patient that actually worsened the condition. In the order in which they are cited above, these are:

drained *Zàng* organ	therapy applied incorrectly	constitutional weakness
liver	vomiting	vacuity of Shén Qì
heart	clearing and moving downward	repletion of Yáng Qì
spleen	cooling and cold	repletion of Yīn Qì
lung	fire	blood dryness
kidney	sweating	vacuity of Yáng Qì

Among these five formulas, Xiè Xīn Tāng (Heart Drain Decoction) is closely related to Gānjiāng Huánglián Huángqín Rénshēn Tāng in the *Shānghánlùn*, except that it contains the single additional ingredient gāncǎo, and the wording of the indications and instructions for preparation differs substantially. Similarly, Xìe Shèn Tāng (Kidney Drain Decoction) is related to Fúlíng Guìzhī Wǔwèi Gāncǎo Tāng from the *Jīnguì yàolüe*, with the addition of the single ingredient shēngjiāng.

All the medicinal ingredients used in these formulas are found in the *Shénnóng běncǎojīng*. We can therefore consider them to be "classical formulas" (經方 *jīngfāng*) in the sense that they are composed in a "classical" style and based on "classical" ingredients, regardless of whether there ever was an original source shared by our text and other "classics" or whether they simply include overlapping information. What is clear is that none of these formulas are literal quotations of any source that Zhāng Zhòngjǐng had access to, unless he merely extracted two of these formulas without the accompanying indications and ignored the rest, which seems highly unlikely.

The attentive reader will have noted a slight, but important difference in my translation of the term 瀉 *xiè* "to drain" in the formula titles between this section and the previous one: The intention of the formulas with 瀉 in the title in the first section was indeed to drain the repletion in each organ, and I have therefore translated them as "liver-draining" or "heart-draining," etc., as a complement in each case to a related "supplementing" 補 formula. By contrast, the formulas in the present section strike me as instead addressing a "drained organ," in the sense of an organ that has been severely exhausted due to inappropriate and invasive medical treatment. I have therefore changed the translation to "Liver Drain," "Heart Drain," etc. The grammar of classical Chinese makes both readings possible.

Section Three

Five Formulas for Supplementing the Five *Zàng* Organs

陶云：經方有救諸勞損病方，亦有五首。然綜觀其要義，蓋不外虛候方加減而已。錄出以備修真之輔，拯人之危也。

然其方意深妙，非俗淺所識，緣諸損候，藏氣互乘，虛實雜錯，藥味寒熱並行，補瀉相參，先聖遺奥，出人意表。

漢晉以還，諸名醫輩，張機、衛氾［汎］、華元化、吳普、皇甫玄晏、支法師、葛稚川、范將軍等，皆當代名賢，咸師式此湯液經法，愍救疾苦，造福含靈。其間增減，雖各擅其異，或致新效，似亂舊經，而其旨趣，仍方圓之規矩也。

Táo [Hóngjǐng] states: Among the classical formulas, there are the those that rescue from the various illnesses of taxation injury, and there are also five of them. This being so, when we look at the key principle underlying all of them, they are merely modifications of formulas for vacuity signs, and nothing more. I have written them out to provide assistance in the cultivation of Perfection, and to bring people back from the precipice of grave danger.

And yet, the meaning of these formulas is profound and subtle, and hence not something that shallow minds can comprehend. Following along with the various signs of injury, the *zàng* organs' Qì exploit each other, vacuity and repletion become intermixed, among the medicinal flavors hot and cold act simultaneously, and supplementing and draining join hands. The relics left behind by the sages from the past are enigmatic and go far beyond the superficial limitations of what people are able to project into the future.

Ever since the Hàn and Jìn dynasties, the various famous physicians, Zhāng Jī, Wèi Xùn, Huà Tuó, Wú Pǔ, Huángfǔ Mì, Zhī Fǎcún, Gě Hóng, Fàn Wāng, etc., all the famous men of virtue of our times, every teacher has emulated these classical methods of decoctions to compassionately save people from illness and suffering and to bestow blessings on all sentient beings. Even though their modifications each excel in the differences that set them apart and may bring about new efficacy, seeming to revolutionize the old classics, yet their ultimate goal still lines up squarely with the old standards.

養生補肝湯

治肝虛筋極，腹中堅澼，大便秘塞方：

蜀椒（汗）	一升
桂心	三兩
韭葉（切）	一把
芍藥	三兩
芒硝	半斤
胡麻油	一升

上六味，以水五升，先煮椒、桂、韭葉、芍藥，取得二升，去滓，納芒硝於內，待消已，即停火。將麻油傾入，乘熱，急以桑枝三枚，各長尺許，不住手攪，令與藥和合為度。共得三升，溫分三服，一日盡之。

Yǎng Shēng Bǔ Gān Tāng
(Life-Nurturing Liver-Supplementing Decoction)

A formula to treat vacuity of the liver with "sinew extreme," hardening and *pì* Afflux in the abdomen, and constipation:

shǔjiāo ([mix-fried until they] sweat)	1 *shēng*
guìxīn	3 *liǎng*
jiǔyè (chopped)	1 handful
sháoyào	3 *liǎng*
mángxiāo	0.5 *jīn*
sesame oil	1 *shēng*

Of the six ingredients above, first use 5 *shēng* of water to decoct the shǔjiāo, guìxīn, jiǔyè, and sháoyào, until reduced to 2 *shēng*. Remove the dregs, add the mángxiāo, and wait until it is dissolved, then stop the flame. Pour in the sesame oil and, taking advantage of the heat, quickly use three mulberry twigs, each about a *chǐ* long, to stir without stopping until all the medicinals are blended completely. Altogether you will obtain 3 *shēng*. Take this warm, divided into three doses, using it all up within one day.

Translator's Note

"Sinew Extreme" is my literal translation of the term 筋極. This term is explained in the *Bèijí qiānjīn yàofāng* 《備急千金要方》 (vol. 11 on the liver) in this way:

夫六極者，天氣通於肺，地氣通於咽，風氣應於肝，雷氣動於心，穀氣感於脾，雨氣潤於腎。六經為川，腸胃為海，九竅為水注之氣，所以竅應於五臟，五臟邪傷，則六腑生極，故曰五臟六極也。。。凡筋極者主肝也，肝應筋，筋與肝合，肝有病從筋生。

The Six Extremes: Heaven's Qì flows through the lung, while Earth's Qì flows through the throat. Wind Qì resonates with the liver, thunder Qì stirs the heart, grain Qì affects the spleen, and rain Qì moistens the kidney. The six channels constitute the rivers, the intestines and stomach constitute the sea, and the nine orifices constitute the Qì of water pouring. Therefore, the orifices resonate with the five zàng *organs, and when the five* zàng *organs are damaged by evil, then the six* fǔ *organs generate the extremes. Thus, we call them the Six Extremes of the five* zàng *organs... Always, Sinew Extreme indicates the liver. The liver resonates with the sinews, and the sinews and the liver are a perfect match. The liver has illness that is engendered from the sinews.*

In the following volume on the gallbladder, Sūn Sīmiǎo describes Sinew Extreme as one of the Six Extremes and as manifesting with "hypertonicity, hardening and distention in the lower abdomen, heart pain, cold in the knees, and pain in all the bones and joints of the four limbs"「筋極則拘攣，小腹堅脹，心痛，膝寒冷，四肢骨節皆痛疼。」.

In the present text, the following formulas similarly associate one of these Extremes each with the associated *zàng* organ: The heart with Vessel Extreme, the spleen with Flesh Extreme, the lung with Qì Extreme, and the kidney with *jīng* Essence Extreme. This list is almost literally identical with Sūn Sīmiǎo's, with the exception that Sūn splits the Extreme associated with the lung into two, into "Qì Extreme" and "Lung Extreme," and refers to the Extreme associated with the kidney as "Bone Extreme," instead of the term "Essence Extreme" used in the present text.

It is interesting that the first, and to my knowledge earliest, list of these Six Extremes as critical medical conditions is found in Cháo Yuánfāng's 巢元方 *Zhūbìng yuánhòu lùn* 《諸病源候論》:

六極者，一曰氣極，令人內虛，五臟不足，邪氣多，正氣少，不欲言。二曰血極，令人無顏色，眉毛墮落，忽忽喜忘。三曰筋極，令人數轉筋，十指爪甲皆痛，苦倦不能久立。四曰骨極，令人酸削，齒苦痛，手足煩疼，不可以立，不欲行動。五曰肌極，令人羸瘦無潤澤，飲食不生肌膚。六曰精極，令人少氣噏噏然內虛，五臟氣不足，發毛落，悲傷喜忘。

The Six Extremes are: One, Qì Extreme, which causes internal vacuity in the person, insufficiency in the five zàng *organs, an increase of evil Qì and a decrease of righteous Qì, and a reluctance to speak; two, Blood Extreme, which causes a lack of color in the person, loss of eyebrow hair, and confusion and forgetfulness; three, Sinew Extreme, which causes frequent twisting of the sinews in the person, pain in all the ten finger nails, and severe fatigue and inability to stand for a long time; four, Bone Extreme, which causes extreme soreness in the person, severe pain in the teeth, vexing pain in the hands and feet, inability to stand up, and reluctance to move and walk; five, Flesh Extreme, which causes marked emaciation and lack of moisture and luster in the person, and failure to engender flesh and skin from eating and drinking; and six, Essence Extreme, which causes scantiness of breath in the person, belabored breathing, and internal vacuity, insufficiency of Qì in the five* zàng *organs, loss of hair on the head, and great sorrow and forgetfulness.*

The fact that the concept of the Six Extremes is, at least to my knowledge, not found in any earlier texts and is also quoted in the

Ishimpō as coming from the *Zhūbìng yuánhòu lùn*, strongly suggests that at least this section of the *Fǔxíngjué* must have been composed AFTER these two publications from the seventh century.

For an explanation on *pì* Afflux, see my note on page 129.

調神補心湯

治心勞脈極，心中煩悸，神識慌惚方：

旋覆花（一方作牡丹皮四兩，當從）	一升
栗子（打，去殼）	十二枚
蔥葉	十四莖
豉（一方作山茰肉，當從）	半斤
梔子（打）	十四枚
人參（切）	三兩

上六味，以清酒四升，水六升，煮取三升，溫分三服，日三。

Tiáo Shén Bǔ Xīn Tāng
(Spirit-Attuning Heart-Supplementing Decoction)

A formula to treat heart taxation and Vessel Extreme, vexing palpitations in the heart, and mental confusion:

xuánfùhuā (an [alternate version of this] formula calls for 4 *liǎng* of mǔdānpí instead. Follow that!)	1 *shēng*
lìzǐ (broken into pieces, husks removed)	12 nuts
cōngyè	14 stalks
dàndòuchǐ (another [version of this] formula calls for shānyúròu. Follow that!)	0.5 *jīn*
zhīzǐ (broken into pieces)	14 fruits
rénshēn (chopped)	3 *liǎng*

Decoct the six ingredients above in 4 *shēng* of clear rice wine and 6 *shēng* of water until reduced to 3 *shēng*. Take warm, divided into three doses, three times a day.

Translator's Note

According to Sūn Sīmiǎo, Vessel Extreme is the third of the Six Extremes and associated with the following constellation of symptoms:

脉極則顏色苦青，逆意，喜恍惚失氣狀似悲泣之後，苦舌强咽喉乾，寒熱惡風不可動，不嗜食，苦眩，喜怒妄言。

...a severe green-blue facial complexion, being contrarian in one's intentions, a tendency to absentmindedness, loss of Qì, and an appearance as if after having shed tears of grief, suffering from a rigid tongue and dry throat, cold and heat and aversion to wind to the point of being unable to move, no craving for food, severe dizziness, and a tendency to forgetfulness and haphazard speech.

建中補脾湯

治脾虛肉極，羸瘦如柴，腹中拘急，四肢無力方：

甘草（炙）	二兩
大棗（去核）	十二枚
生薑（切）	三兩
黃飴	一升
芍藥	六兩
桂枝	二兩

上六味，以水七升，煮取三升。去滓，納飴，更上火，令消已。溫服一升，日盡之。

Jiàn Zhōng Bǔ Pí Tāng
(Center-Building and Spleen-Supplementing Decoction)

A formula for treating vacuity of the spleen with Flesh Extreme, marked emaciation so they look like sticks and bones, hypertonicity in the abdomen, and lack of strength in the four limbs:

gāncǎo (mix-fried)	2 *liǎng*
dàzǎo	12 pieces
shēngjiāng (chopped)	3 *liǎng*
yítáng	1 *shēng*
sháoyào	6 *liǎng*
guìzhī	2 *liǎng*

Decoct the six ingredients above in 7 *shēng* of water until reduced to 3 *shēng*. Remove the dregs, add the malt sugar, and place it back on the flame until it is completely dissolved. Take 1 *shēng* per dose warm, using everything up in a day.

Translator's Note

Sūn Sīmiǎo lists Flesh Extreme as the sixth type of Extreme and describes it in very dire terms:

六肉極則發疰如得擊，不復言，甚者至死復生，衆醫所不能治。

Six: Flesh Extreme. Results in an outbreak of Influx Disease as if the person had been beaten, not recovering their ability to speak, in severe cases getting to the point of dying and returning to life, a condition that multitudes of doctors are unable to treat.

This formula is almost exactly identical with Xiǎo Jiàn Zhōng Tāng (Minor Center-Building Decoction) from the *Shānghánlùn*, except that it calls for 2 *liǎng* of guìzhī instead of 3.

寧氣補肺湯

治肺虛氣極，煩熱汗出，口舌渴燥方：

麥門冬	二升
五味子	二升
白截漿	五升
芥子	半升
旋覆花	一兩
竹葉	三把

上六味，但以白截漿共煮，取得三升，分三服，日盡之。

Níng Qì Bǔ Fèi Tāng
(Qì-Calming Lung-Supplementing Decoction)

A formula to treat vacuity of the lung with Qì Extreme, vexing heat and sweating, and thirst and dryness in the mouth and tongue:

màiméndōng	2 *shēng*
wǔwèizǐ	2 *shēng*
báizàijiāng	5 *shēng*
jièzǐ	0.5 *shēng*
xuánfùhuā	1 *liǎng*
zhúyè	3 handfuls

Of the six ingredients above, decoct everything together in only the fermented rice drink (báizàijiāng) until reduced to 3 *shēng* and divide into three doses. Use it all up in a day.

Translator's Note

According to Sūn Sīmiǎo, Qì Extreme is the first of the Six Extremes, while Lung Extreme is listed separately as the second of the Six Extremes. Here is the original citation from volume 38 of the *Bèijí qiānjīn yàofāng*:

一氣極則多寒痺，腹痛，喘息，驚恐，
頭痛。二肺極則寒痺，腰痛，心下堅有積聚，
小便不利，手足不仁。

One: Qì Extreme. Results in increased cold bì *Impediment, abdominal pain, panting, panic and fear, and headache. Two: Lung Extreme. Results in cold* bì *Impediment, pain in the lumbar area, hardening and presence of accumulations and gatherings below the heart, inhibited urination, and numbness of the hands and feet.*

固元補腎湯

治腎虛精極，遺精失溺，氣乏無力，不可轉動，唾血咯血方：

地黃（切）	
王瓜根（切）	各三兩
苦酒	一升
甘草（炙）	
薤白	四兩
乾薑（切）	二兩

上方六味，以苦酒合井泉水五升煮之，取得三升，每服一升，一日盡之。

Gù Yuán Bŭ Shèn Tāng
(Origin-Securing Kidney-Supplementing Decoction)

A formula to treat vacuity in the kidney with Essence Extreme, seminal emission and urinary incontinence, Qì exhaustion and lack of strength, inability to turn from side to side, and spitting up and coughing up of blood:

dìhuáng (chopped)	
wángguāgēn (chopped)	3 *liăng* each
kŭjiŭ	1 *shēng*
gāncăo (mix-fried)	
xièbái	4 *liăng*
gānjiāng (chopped)	2 *liăng*

Decoct the six ingredients from the formula above in a combination of the soured rice wine with 5 *shēng* of well water, until reduced to 3 *shēng*. Take 1 *shēng* per dose, using everything up in a single day.

Translator's Note

Sūn Sīmiăo's list of the Six Extremes does not include Essence Extreme but instead has "Bone Extreme," which is described with these symptoms:

五骨極則肢節厥逆，黃膽消渴，癰疽妄發，重病浮腫如水病狀。

> *Five: Bone Extreme. Results in counter-current reversal in the limb joints, yellow gallbladder dispersion thirst, welling-abscesses and flat-abscesses erupting haphazardly, and repeatedly falling ill with floating swelling like water disease.*

As already mentioned above, Cháo Yuánfāng describes the manifestations of Essence Extreme as "scantiness of breath in the person, belabored breathing, and internal vacuity, insufficiency of Qì in the five *zàng* organs, loss of hair on the head, and great sorrow and forgetfulness."

陶云：經云：毒藥攻邪，五菜為充，五果為助，五穀為養，五畜為益。爾乃大湯之設。今所錄者，皆小湯耳。若欲作大湯者，補肝湯內加羊肝，補心加雞心，補脾加牛肉，補肺加犬肺，補腎加豬腎，各一具，即成也。

Táo [Hóngjǐng] states: According to the Classic, toxic medicinals attack evils, the five vegetables provide fullness, the five fruits provide assistance, the five grains provide nourishment, and the five farm animals provide additional benefit. This then is how you build large decoctions. What is recorded in the present text are all small decoctions. if you want to turn them into large decoctions, add mutton liver to the decoction for supplementing the liver, chicken heart to supplement the heart, beef flesh to supplement the spleen, dog lung to supplement the lung, and pig kidney to supplement the kidney, 1 piece each, and that makes it complete.

Translator's Note

The quotation from the "Classic" refers to *Sùwèn* 22:

> 毒藥攻邪，五穀為養，五果為助，五畜為益，五菜為充，氣味合而服之，以補精益氣。

> *Toxic medicinals attack evils, the five grains provide nourishment, the five fruits provide assistance, the five farm animals provide additional benefit, and the five vegetables provide fullness. By consuming these with the Qì and flavors well-matched, we supplement* jīng *Essence and boost Qì.*

According to the famous *Nèijīng* commentator Wáng Bīng 王冰, the five vegetables are "mallow, pulse leaves, scallion, garlic-chives, onion" (葵、藿、韭、薤、葱), the five fruits are "peach, plum, apricot, chestnut, and jujube" (桃、李、杏、栗、棗), the five grains are "non-glutinous rice, adzuki bean, wheat/barley, soybean, and broomcorn millet" (粳米、小豆、麥、大豆、黃黍), and the five farm animals are "cow, sheep/goat, dog, pig, chicken" (牛羊犬豕雞).

This concludes the third major section of our source text *Fŭxíngjué zàngfŭ yòngyàofă*. After the 24 major and minor formulas for draining and supplementing each of the five *zàng* organs in the first section, with four extra formulas for the heart, then the five organ-drain formulas and five organ-supplementing formulas, we now arrive at a very different layer of the text, which is concerned not with formulas but with individual medicinals, their classification into flavors, and the specific actions associated with each. It is unfortunate that Chinese authors in traditional times rarely cite their sources and that other sources, like the Japanese *Ishimpō* 醫心方, which do cite their sources, do not include this information. This makes it impossible for us today to track this information further back and we are left with the vague sense that this text was compiled after Táo Hóngjĭng's lifetime and before the Dūnhuáng 敦煌 caves were closed in the early Sòng period. So, although a creation of early medieval China, it may very well contain earlier material."

Section Four

The Five Flavors and Twenty-Five Medicinals

4.1

Introduction and Essay

陶隱居云：依神農本經及桐君採藥錄，上中下三品之藥，凡三百六十五味，以應周天之度，四時八節之氣。商有聖相伊尹，撰湯液經三卷，為方，亦三百六十首：上品上藥，為服食補益方者百二十者；中品中藥，為療疾祛邪之方，亦百十十首；下品毒藥，為殺蟲辟邪之方，亦百二十首。凡共三百六十首也。實萬代醫家之規範，蒼生護命之大寶也。

今檢錄常情需用者六十首，備山中預防災疾之用耳。檢用諸藥之要者，可默契經方之旨焉。經云：在天成象，在地成形，天有五氣，化生五味，五味之變，不可勝數。今者約列二十五種，以明五行互含之跡，以明五味變化之用，如左。

Hermit Táo [Hóngjǐng] states: According to the *Divine Farmer's Classic of Materia Medica* and *Lord Tóng's Record of Picking Medicinals*, the three grades of medicinals—upper, middle, and lower—altogether comprise 365 substances, thereby resonating with the complete 360-degree circle of the universe and with the Qì of the Four Seasons and Eight Nodes. In the Shāng dynasty, there was the sagely minister Yī Yǐn who composed a *Decoction Classic* in three volumes, consisting of formulas, also with 360 entries. The upper grade with the upper medicinals consisted of formulas for alchemical foods and supplementing and boosting, of which there were 120. The middle grade with middle medicinals consisted of formulas for curing illness and driving away evils, of which there were also 120. The lower grade with toxic medicinals consisted of formulas for killing worms and warding off evils, of which there were also 120. So in total there were altogether 360 entries. Truly, this has been the standard for myriad generations of physicians and the great treasure for protecting the life of all the people.

At present, here is a collection of sixty often-used formulas, to be ready for use in the mountains as a precaution against natural calamities and illness. As we examine the essence of how the various medicinals are used, we can form an invisible bond with the aim of the classical formulas through them. As the Classic states, "in Heaven to complete the archetype, on earth to complete the form." Heaven has the Five Qì, which transform to engender the Five Flavors. The alterations of the Five Flavors are too many to count.

The present text arranges twenty-five kinds, to bring to light the visible traces of how the Five Agents contain each other, to bring to light the applications of the transformations and alterations of the Five Flavors, as [is expressed] below:

Translator's Note

The closest source I have been able to track down for the quote from the "Classic" appears to be the *Zhōu Yì Xìcí* 《周易繫辭》(Appendix on the *Yìjīng*), one of the famous commentaries on the *Yìjīng* traditionally attributed to Confucius. The passage there says: 「在天成象，在地成形，變化見矣。」 "In Heaven to complete the archetype, on earth to complete the form, becoming manifest in the transformations and alterations."

And a nerdy note is in order here, because it is just too beautiful to ignore: The English term "contain," which I have reluctantly used to translate the Chinese character 含, simply does not do it justice. The character literally means "to hold something in the mouth," sometimes in the specific context of the piece of jade or similar ritual object placed in the mouth of a dead body before burial. As such, it includes the notions of "to embody," and both "to support" and "to restrain." I could not think of a more perfect way to conceptualize the mutual interactions of the Five Agents that includes both the 生 *shēng* (generate) and the 剋 *kè* (control) cycles.

In terms of the format of this entire section, it is not clear whether the entire section is meant as a statement by Táo Hóngjǐng or whether only the first section is, since classical Chinese does not contain punctuation marks, and thus also no opening and closing quotation marks. I have followed the contemporary Chinese editors of the text in reading this all as a statement by Táo Hóngjǐng, but the discerning reader does need to keep in mind that that is a decision made by modern editors more than a thousand years after the original composition of the text.

Lastly, I would like to draw the reader's attention to the seemingly innocuous phrase "for use in the mountains as a precaution." This is a direct reflection of Táo Hóngjǐng's — or rather, his impersonator's — primary interest in and reason for involvement with this text, which he already stated at the beginning: as the first step and necessary foundation, a safeguard to prepare for the key goal of his life, which was spiritual and alchemical transformation in the pursuit of immortality. Like Sūn Sīmiǎo 孫思邈, Gě Hóng 葛洪, and so many other medical authors of the early medieval period, Táo was not a professionally practicing physician but a member of the literate elite who had withdrawn to the mountains as a hermit and focused his efforts, especially in his later life, on texts, knowledge, and practices that would strike us modern readers as utterly foreign and esoteric. As we read their texts and extract information to use in contemporary clinical practice, it is important to keep this original historical context in mind, especially in the evaluation and categorization of medicinal substances, and here formulas as well, into the three grades of upper, middle, and lower.

味辛皆屬木，桂為之主，椒為火，薑為土，細辛為金，□□為水。

味鹹皆屬火，旋覆花為之主，大黃為木，澤瀉為土，厚朴為金，硝石為水。

味甘皆屬土，人參為之主，甘草為木，大棗為火，麥冬為金，茯苓為水。

味酸皆屬金，五味為之主，枳實為木，豉為火，芍藥為土，薯蕷為水。

味苦皆屬水，地黃為之主，黃芩為木，黃連為火，白朮為土，竹味為水。

此二十五味，為諸藥之精，多療五臟六腑內損諸病，學者當深契焉。

[Substances that are] acrid in flavor all belong to Wood. Guìzhī constitutes their ruler, [shǔ]jiāo constitutes Fire, gān/shēngjiāng constitutes Earth, xìxīn constitutes Metal, and □□ constitutes Water.

[Substances that are] salty in flavor all belong to Fire. Xuánfùhuā constitutes their ruler, dàhuáng constitutes Wood, zéxiè constitutes Earth, hòupò constitutes Metal, and xiāoshí constitutes Water.

[Substances that are] sweet in flavor all belong to Earth. Rénshēn constitutes their ruler, gāncǎo constitutes Wood, dàzǎo constitutes Fire, màiméndōng constitutes Metal, and fúlíng constitutes Water.

[Substances that are] sour in flavor all belong to Metal. Wǔwèizǐ constitutes their ruler, zhǐshí constitutes Wood, dàndòuchǐ constitutes Fire, sháoyào constitutes Earth, and shǔyù constitutes Water.

[Substances that are] bitter in flavor all belong to Water. Dìhuáng constitutes their ruler, huángqín constitutes Wood, huánglián constitutes Fire, báizhú constitutes Earth, and zhǔyè constitutes Water.

These twenty-five flavors constitute the Essence of all the various medicinals and, in most cases, cure all the various illnesses of internal injury in the five *zàng* and six *fǔ* organs. In studying these, we must form a deep bond with them.

Translator's Note

There is an unfortunate lacuna in the first line of this section in the original text, namely the Water medicinal in the category of the acrid flavor. The name of the medicinal is missing in the two major transcriptions of the *Fǔxíngjué*, the one by Zhāng Dàcháng and the one done by his disciples. Contemporary teachers of this material tend to insert fùzǐ here as the medicinal in question but this addition should be treated with caution.

4.2

Chart

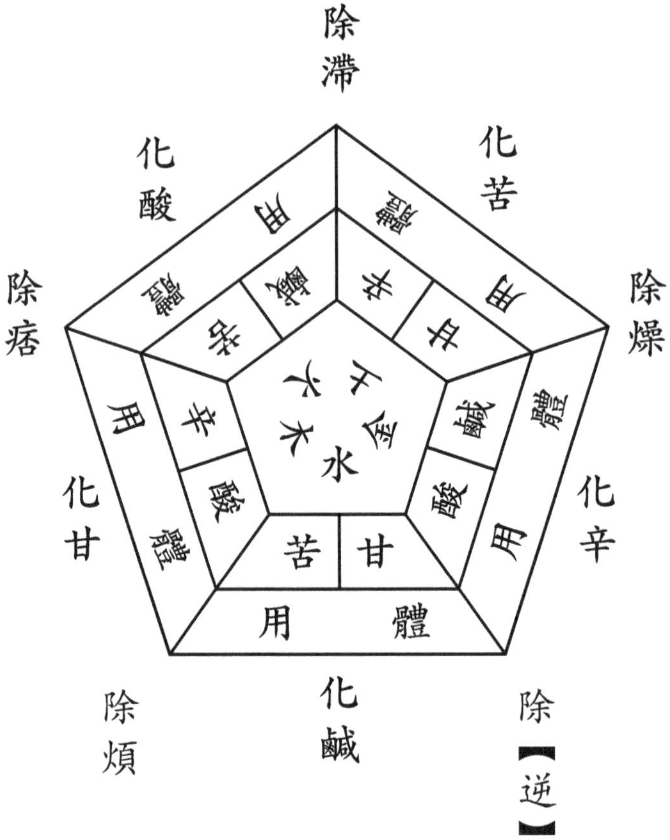

右

陰退為瀉
其數六水數也

陽進為補
其數七火數也

左

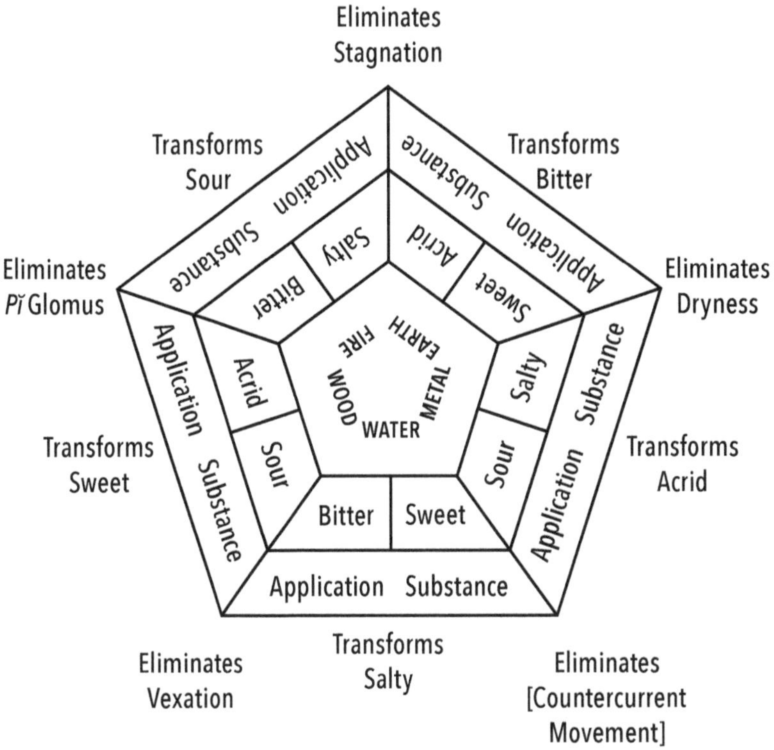

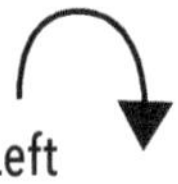

Left

Yáng advancing
causes supplementation.
Its number is seven,
which is the
number of Fire.

Right

Yin retreating
causes draining.
Its number is six,
which is the
number of Water

Translator's Note

Please be aware that in the critical editions of the text this chart does not have a title, which means that the medical historians in China who created these editions did not consider any title to have been a part of the original manuscript. The manuscript versions from the 1960s and 1970s by Zhāng Dàchāng and his disciples have varying titles, of which this one in the version by Liú Déxìng 劉德興 from 1974 seems to be the earliest: "Chart for matching the ruler, minister, assistants, and envoys, supplementing and draining, substance and application, and changes in the essential methods for using medicinals for the five *zàng* organs." The complete absence or variations in any title attached to the chart in these manuscripts is incontrovertible proof that any title that associates it with the lost *Tāngyèjīng* is a modern addition and can therefore not be used to argue that this chart comes from that text or dates from the Hàn dynasty. In particular, the label 《湯液經法圖》 ("Chart of the Classical Methods of Decoctions") is very clearly a modern addition.

經云：主於補瀉者為君，數量同於君而非主故為臣，從於佐監者為佐使。

The Classic states: "[Substances] that are in charge of supplementing and draining constitute the rulers; [substances] that are identical in quantity to the ruler but are not in charge constitute the ministers; [substances that] follow to assist the supervisors constitute the assistants and envoys."

陶隱居曰：此圖乃湯液經法盡要之妙，學者能諳於此，醫道畢矣。

The hermit Táo [Hóngjǐng] states: This chart indeed [reflects] the utterly significant subtlety of the classical methods of decoctions. When those who study them are able to know them by heart, their Dào of medicine has reached its destination!

Translator's Note

I have been unable to track down the original source of the "classical methods" in the statement above. Given that some of the other quotations of the "Classic" in this text are less than literal, this may have to remain an unsolved mystery.

Section Five

External Contractions of Celestial Movements

5.1

Introduction

弘景曰：外感天行，經方之治，有二旦、六神大小等湯。昔南陽張機，依此諸方，撰為《傷寒論》一部，療治明悉，後學咸尊奉之。

山林僻居，倉卒難防外感之疾，日數傳變，生死往往在三五日間，豈可疏忽。若能深明此數方者，則庶無蹈險之虞也。今亦錄而識之。

[Táo] Hóngjǐng states: Among the classical formulas for external contractions of celestial movements, there are the two Dawning and six Spirit decoctions, in major and minor grades. In the past Zhāng Jī from Nányáng relied on these various formulas to compose the *Treatise on Cold Damage* in one section. Given how incisive and comprehensive these treatments are, later students all revere them.

Those of us who dwell secluded in mountains and forests are all of sudden confronted with critical illnesses of external contraction that are difficult to avoid. With numerous transmissions and changes each day, life and death are often on the line within only three to five days. How could we possibly be careless about this! If we are able to deeply understand these several formulas, then we might just avoid the worrisome prospect of this risk. At present I have also recorded them and committed them to memory.

Translator's Note

There are two significant details in the way I have translated characters or phrases that differ from the standard practice: First, I want to look at the phrase at the beginning of Táo Hóngjǐng's quote, namely the expression 外感天行 *wàigǎn tiānxíng*, which I have translated as "external contractions of celestial movements." The two characters 天行 *tiānxíng* first started appearing together in medieval texts, indicating that this combination is not an ancient term or concept. Following current convention, this phrase tends to be translated as "epidemic" or even as "seasonal" in technical medical literature. According to the Merriam-Webster dictionary, however, an epidemic is defined as "an outbreak of disease that spreads quickly and affects many individuals at the same time."[1] This definition is not in accordance with the meaning of the Chinese term in the context of this text and the actual formulas, many of which are used for chronic or both chronic and acute illnesses. I suggest that we think of this expression here in a more literal sense as "activity/movement in Heaven/sky," which actually works quite well even though it sounds a bit stilted at first sight. What we can say is that this "external contraction of celestial movements" means that the formulas are meant to be used to help people who have been affected by movement in the sky/Heaven and that this celestial movement is external to them.

Second, I translate 旦 *dàn* when it occurs in the name of Major and Minor Yáng and Yīn Dàn Tāng not as a noun "dawn," but as a verb "dawning," which gives us "Dawning of Yīn" and "Dawning of Yáng." Grammatically, this is more likely here in part because of the consistent balance of Yīn and Yáng formulas in the present text. In other words, it is unlikely, given this balance, that there would be two formulas associated with dawn, in the meaning of the literal dawn in the early morning of the day, without there also being two formulas for dusk. The translation of *dàn* as "dawning" further emphasizes that we are not dealing with the literal dawn but rather with the metaphorical concept of the light of the sun just barely above the horizon, or with the process of the sun rising above the horizon and becoming visible, as expressed by the etymology of the character: a depiction of the sun just above the horizon. Metaphorically, this "dawning" means the very beginning of something, in this case the beginning of Yīn and the beginning of Yáng. As such, we can see that Yáng Dawning Decoction refers to the beginning of Yáng, which correlates with the time of dawn, while Yīn Dawning Decoction refers to the beginning of Yīn, which correlates with the time of dusk. The definition of *dàn* in the *Shuōwén jiězì* dictionary from the Hàn period actually explains the character as identical with 明 *míng* "brightness," and literally, a

[1] See https://www.merriam-webster.com/dictionary/epidemic.

combination of the sun and the moon. In our attempt to understand the intended action of these formulas in a concrete clinical context, this distinction may prove helpful as we contemplate the meaning of "Yīn dawning" versus "Yáng dawning."

Lastly, a note on this section is in order. Medical historians are largely in agreement that the formulas in this section have a genuine classical feel to them. In addition, they are very closely related to *Shānghánlùn* formulas. Though we cannot know whether these formulas pre-dated the *Shānghánlùn* or vice versa, we can say that this grouping of *Liù Shén* and *Èr Dàn* formulas share a common ancestor with the *Shānghánlùn*.

On the basis of this close relationship between the formulas in this section and the *Shānghánlùn*, medical historian Wáng Shūmín argues: "From my extensive comparison of the remedies above, I have established that the major formulae in Zhang Zhongjing's *Shanghan lun* and the *erdan* and *liushen* formulae attributed to *Tangye* have common elements: they either share titles, or have different titles yet the same ingredients; some of them differ only in the addition or reduction of some ingredients. On the basis of this evidence, I have concluded that *Shanghan lun* is a pharmacological text that has inherited and evolved the canonical recipes of *erdan* and *liushen*."[2] What is essential to keep in mind here is the fact that the *Fǔxíngjué* is not identical with the *Tāngyèjīng* and, while probably containing formulas that were ancestral to Zhāng Zhòngjǐng's work, cannot be read as a Hàn dynasty text. The compilation of the various textual layers, the introductory and concluding comments, and most likely a large portion of even the formulas or other textual layers, clearly date to a time after Táo Hóngjǐng's death.

[2] See Vivienne Lo and Christopher Cullen, eds., *Medieval Chinese Medicine*, p. 340.

Commentary by Sharon Weizenbaum

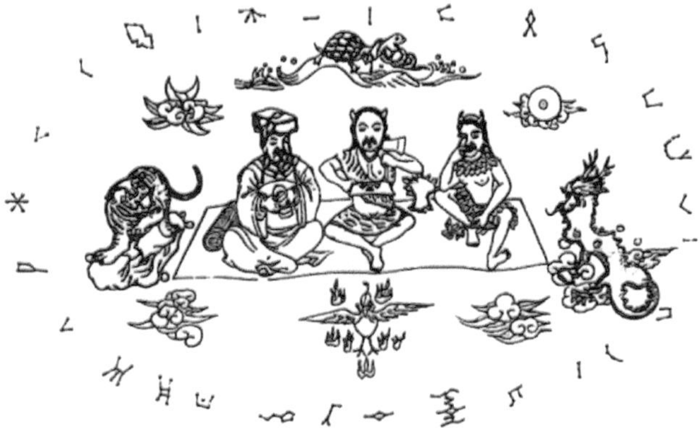

Huangdi, Shennong and Fuxi, surrounded by the Guardian Spirits of the Four Directions, the Sun, the Moon and the 28 Lunar Mansions.

The two Dawning (二旦 *èr dàn*) and six Spirit (六神 *liù shén*) formulas are one of the most important and clinically interesting sections in the *Fǔxíngjué*. Given that these formulas' names and ingredients closely match some that are found in the *Shānghán zábìnglùn*, their origin is likely more ancient than the material in the rest of the *Fǔxíngjué*, perhaps even dating to the Hàn Dynasty (206 BCE – 220 CE).

A bit of background to explain my interest in these formulas: Around the year 2005, after almost 25 years of practice, I became drawn to classical formulas. The formula architecture and effectiveness of these formulas set them apart from more modern formulas. I diligently read the *Shānghán zábìnglùn*, looking for a thread of meaning or principles but found it mostly impenetrable. I understood the formulas in a this-for-this and that-for-that kind of way but couldn't find any sense of the text's unifying structure. I studied with various classical formula teachers in China and the United States.

Though I learned a lot about classifying and utilizing the formulas, I was still not seeing the one integrative essence.

In 2007, I finally had an insight that completely shifted my understanding of the text. I heard a quote from the famous Chinese doctor Liú Lìhóng 劉力紅: "It's all about tracking the Yáng." In a moment, I understood the text as describing the circular dynamics of Yáng, or the life-force, in the body. In my imagination, I saw the sun's relative movement around the earth as connected to the circulation of the life force or Yáng (from here the life force Yáng) in our bodies. It then made sense that what we in English have come to know as the "Six Conformations" or "Six Levels" but what in Chinese is known as the 六經 *liùjīng* does not express relative depths in the body from Tàiyáng on the outside to Juéyīn at the deepest level, as I had been taught. Instead, these *liùjīng* could be expressing movements of the life-force Yáng within our bodies as directed by movements of the heavens above. Suddenly the text and the formulas within it made great sense to me! The time of this insight was such a revelatory moment for me. I felt like Helen Keller finally connecting the feeling of water with her teacher's finger spelling. It was the dawning of meaning. Since that time, I have been working with and teaching classical formulas from this vantage point. As time went on, I found that others had similar insights and wrote about them in various inspiring ways (such as Péng Zǐyì's article on the circular dynamics of ancient Chinese medicine in *The Lantern*).

When I first saw the section of the *Fǔxíngjué* that talks about the six Spirit and two Dawning formulas, it made immediate sense to me that this was an expanded expression of the circular dynamics I had come to see as the core of my approach to the *Shānghánlùn* and East Asian medicine in general.

As I do in my work with and teaching of the *Shānghán zábìnglùn*, I am applying my lens to this material here, always with a critical awareness that my narrative about it is not the only correct way to look at it. That said, when I interpret texts, especially classical texts,

I do make sure that my interpretation is consistent with the text and other related texts and, more importantly, that it adds to clarity and clinical relevance. When my interpretation causes complex information to simplify and fall into place, I always feel I'm onto something. As Albert Einstein said, "Everything should be made as simple as possible, but not simpler."

This section of the *Fǔxíngjué* describes eight formulas, for which there are major and minor expressions. I suggest that we see these formulas as tools to re-establish the patient's right relationship with the celestial movements. The first four of these Six Spirits represent the traditional Chinese guardian spirits of the four directions (east, south, west, and north, respectively) as well as groupings of stars in the four quadrants of the sky. These are the Green-Blue Dragon, White Tiger, Vermilion Bird, and Dark Warrior. Among the last two, one represents the central axis around the north star, which is called the Hooking Array, and one represents the joining of fire and water in the north, called the Soaring Serpent.

What are the celestial movements and how do these movements relate to a human being's physiology and pathology? I would like the reader to consider the image of our life-force Yáng ascending and descending in a circular pathway within our bodies, just as the sun and moon appear to rise and fall around the earth. Imagine that when a body is in harmony with the circular rising and falling of the heavens, there is health. Health is a result of being in right relationship with the guardian spirits of the directions. Imagine that ascending in my body is related to the east's dynamic, where the sun, moon, and stars all ascend continually. Descending in my body is then related to the west's dynamic of celestial orbs setting. Imagine that the proper ascending of the life-force Yáng in my body is the same as being in alignment with the east's guardian spirit, the Green-blue Dragon, and descending in my body is the same as being in right relationship with the west's guardian spirit, the White Tiger. Failing to be in right relationship with a quadrant's guardian spirit means my body's life force Yáng is too slow or too fast in its rising and falling relative to the ascending and descending of the celestial bodies. We could also call this being sick.

I'll go over the spirit formulas for each of the four quadrants, the center, and both the Yīn and Yáng Dawnings separately, to give an overview of their structure and relevance. These formulas are directed at the body to align it with time. Time is kept through the celestial movements. In the *Fǔxíngjué*, the symptoms of each formula presentation are defined as being caused by 天行 *tiānxíng*. This term is sometimes translated as "epidemic" or "contagious," however Wilms and I have chosen to translate it as "celestial movements" because the context is so obviously about the movement of the celestial bodies. We feel that translating it as "epidemic" or "contagious" greatly limits our understanding. We will see that all of the formulas in this section use the flavor and temperature of medicinals to encourage appropriate movement with time, as well as the nature of the herbs, such as their density, lightness, juiciness, hardness, or suppleness.

5.2

The Minor and Major Formulas of the Two Yáng and Yīn Dàn Decoctions

小陽旦湯

治天行發熱，自汗出而惡風，鼻鳴乾嘔者。

桂枝	三兩
芍藥	三兩
生薑（切）	二兩
甘草（炙）	二兩
大棗	十二枚

上方，以水七升，煮取三升，溫服一升。服已，即啜熱粥飯一器，以助藥力，稍令汗出，不可大汗，流漓汗之則病不除也。若不汗出，可隨服之，取瘥止。日三服。

若加飴一升，為正陽旦湯。

Xiǎo Yáng Dàn Tāng
(Minor Yáng-Dawning Decoction)

For treating heat effusion caused by celestial movements, with spontaneous sweating and aversion to wind, noisy breathing from the nose, and dry retching.

guìzhī	3 *liǎng*
sháoyào	3 *liǎng*
shēngjiāng (chopped)	2 *liǎng*
gāncǎo (mix-fried)	2 *liǎng*
dàzǎo	12 pieces

Decoct [the ingredients from] the formula above in 7 *shēng* of water until reduced to 3 *shēng*. Take 1 *shēng* per dose, warm. After you have taken it, eat a bowl of hot rice gruel in order to assist the power of the medicine and gently cause a bit of sweating. You must not induce great sweating! If the sweat is streaming and dripping down, this means that the illness is not eliminated. If there is no sweat coming out, you can follow up with another dose [of the medicine]. Once you have achieved a cure, stop. Take three doses a day.

If you add 1 *shēng* of yítáng, it becomes Zhèng Yáng Dàn Tāng (Straight Yáng Dawning Decoction).

Translator's Note

The difference in wording between the present formula and the formula for Guìzhī Tāng 桂枝湯 (Cinnamon Decoction) in the

Shānghánlùn suggests that neither text was copied from the other and that the two texts are several sources removed from each other. Nevertheless, the instructions about inducing sweating by consuming hot rice gruel but avoiding excessive sweating suggest either a shared ancestor or, more likely, that this formula was inspired by Zhāng Zhòngjǐng's writings. The compound "Yáng Dawning" 陽旦 is found in both the *Shānghánlùn* and the *Jīnguì yàolüe* (in the sections on Tàiyáng disease and women's postpartum conditions, respectively): In the *Shānghánlùn* in the expression "Yáng Dawning Pattern" 陽旦證, it describes a complication after taking Guìzhī Tāng. In the *Jīnguì yàolüe*, a mere reference to Yáng Dàn Tāng is taken by most subsequent medical authors as an alternate name for Guìzhī Tāng or a modification thereof. It is most interesting that the parallel expression "Yīn Dawning" 陰旦 is not found anywhere else in the received medical literature.

Zhèng Yáng Dàn Tāng is a formula found in the *Bèijí qiānjīn yàofāng*, vol. 30, where it is listed as a modification of Yáng Dàn Tāng: "For vacuity taxation and interior tension, Zhèng Yáng Dàn governs it. Simmer it to obtain 2 *shēng*, add 0.5 *jīn* of jiāoyí (malt syrup), and take in two doses." 「虛勞裏急正陽旦主之煎得二升內膠飴半斤為再服。」

This reference to a modification from the *Qiānjīnfāng* suggests that the author of the *Fǔxíngjué* was familiar with that text and compiled it after the publication of the *Qiānjīnfāng* in the seventh century. Of course, it is also possible that both texts share a common ancestor. Given the fact that Sūn Sīmiǎo makes no mention of either the *Tāngyèjīng* or the *Fǔxíngjué* and does not cite this content in any systematic way or even mention its theories on medicinal resonances and categorizations, it is highly unlikely that the influence went in the other direction.

On the other hand, anybody familiar with classical formulas will recognize the close overlap of the formula here with Guìzhī Tāng 桂枝

湯 (Cinnamon Decoction) and Xiǎo Jiàn Zhōng Tāng 小建中湯 (Minor Center-Building Decoction) from the *Shānghánlùn*.

小陰旦湯

治天行身熱汗出，頭目痛，腹中痛，乾嘔下利者。

黃芩	三兩
芍藥	三兩
生薑（切）	二兩
甘草（炙）	二兩
大棗	十二枚

上方，以水七升，煮取三升，溫服一升，日三服。服湯已，如人行三四里時，令病人啜白截漿一器，以助藥力。身熱去自愈也。

Xiǎo Yīn Dàn Tāng
(Minor Yīn-Dawning Decoction

For treating generalized heat and sweating due to celestial movements, with pain in the head and eyes, pain in the abdomen, dry retching, and diarrhea:

huángqín	3 *liǎng*
sháoyào	3 *liǎng*
shēngjiāng (chopped)	2 *liǎng*
gāncǎo (mix-fried)	2 *liǎng*
dàzǎo	12 pieces

Decoct [the ingredients from] the formula above in 7 *shēng* of water until reduced to 3 *shēng*, and take warm, 1 *shēng* per dose, three doses per day. After you have taken the decoction, wait for the length of time that it takes a person to walk three or four *lǐ* and then make the patient drink down 1 bowl of fermented rice drink, in order to assist the power of the medicine. When the generalized heat is gone, this means spontaneous recovery.

大陽旦湯

治凡病汗出不止，氣息惙惙，身勞力怯，惡風涼，腹中拘急，不欲飲食，皆宜此方。若脈虛大者，為更切證也。

黃芪	五兩
人參	
桂枝	
生薑	各三兩
甘草（炙）	二兩
芍藥	六兩
大棗	十二枚
飴	一升

上七味，以水一斗，煮取四升，去滓。納飴上火，令烊已。每服一升，日三夜一服。

Dà Yáng Dàn Tāng
(Major Yáng-Dawning Decoction)

To treat all cases of suffering from sweating that will not stop, with gasping breathing, generalized taxation and physical frailness, aversion to wind and coolness, hypertonicity in the abdomen, and no interest in drinking and eating, this formula is always suitable. If the pulse is vacuous and large, it is even more of a closely fitting pattern.

huángqí	5 *liǎng*
rénshēn	
guìzhī	
shēngjiāng	3 *liǎng* each
gāncǎo (mix-fried)	2 *liǎng*
sháoyào	6 *liǎng*
dàzǎo	12 pieces
yítáng	1 *shēng*

Decoct the first seven ingredients in 1 *dǒu* of water until reduced to 4 *shēng* and remove the dregs. Add the yítáng and place it back on the flame, making it melt completely. Take 1 *shēng* per dose, three times a day and once at night.

大陰旦湯

治凡病頭目眩暈，咽中乾，每喜乾嘔，食不下，心中煩滿，胸脅支痛，往來寒熱方：

柴胡	八兩
人參	
黃芩	
生薑	各三兩
甘草（炙）	二兩
芍藥	四兩
大棗	十二枚
半夏（洗）	一升

上八味，以水一斗二升，煮取六升，去滓，重上火，緩緩煎之，取得三升。溫服一升，日三服。

Dà Yīn Dàn Tāng
(Major Yīn-Dawning Decoction)

A formula to treat all cases of suffering from dizziness in the head and eyes, dryness in the throat, constant tendency to dry retching, inability to get down food, vexation and fullness in the heart, propping pain in the chest and rib-sides, and alternating cold and heat:

cháihú	8 *liǎng*
rénshēn	
huángqín	
shēngjiāng	3 *liǎng* each
gāncǎo (mix-fried)	2 *liǎng*
sháoyào	4 *liǎng*
dàzǎo	12 pieces
bànxià (washed)	1 *shēng*

Decoct the eight ingredients above in 1 *dǒu* and 2 *shēng* of water until reduced to 6 *shēng*. Remove the dregs and return to the flame. Simmer it very gently until reduced to 3 *shēng*. Take warm, 1 *shēng* per dose, three doses a day.

Translator Note

The similarity between this formula and the formula for Xiǎo Cháihú Tāng (Minor Bupleurum Decoction) in the *Shānghánlùn* is striking and suggests either that the author(s) of the *Fǔxíngjué* copied Zhāng Zhòngjǐng's text or that the two texts share a common source. For readers who do not have the entire *Shānghánlùn* memorized, the indications for Xiǎo Cháihú Tāng are: "For wind strike after five or six days of cold damage, with alternating cold and heat, bitter fullness in the chest and rib-sides, refusal to speak and no interest in drinking and eating, heart vexation and tendency to retching, possibly vexation in the chest but no retching, possibly thirst, possibly pain in the abdomen, possibly *pǐ* Glomus and hardness below the rib-sides, possibly palpitations below the heart and inhibited urination, possibly no thirst and mild generalized heat, and possibly cough, Xiǎo Cháihú Tāng rules." The formula ingredients are the same, with slightly different proportions, except that sháoyào is missing.

Commentary by Sharon Weizenbaum

The fifth major section of the *Fǔxíngjué* begins with the Major and Minor Yīn and Yáng Dawning formulas, *Dàn Tāng* 旦湯. These are the Dawning of Yáng formulas and the Dawning of Yīn formulas.

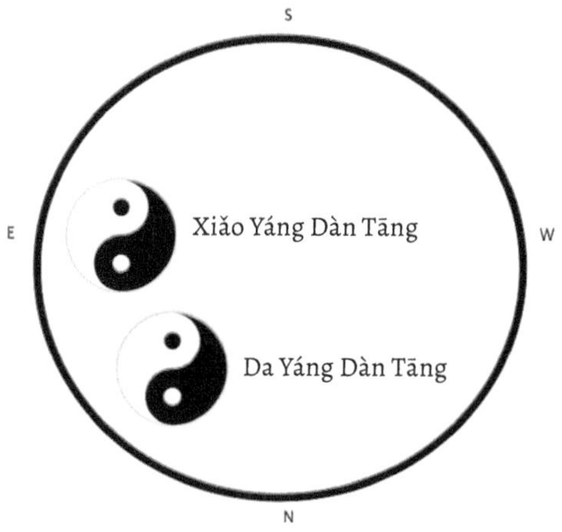

The Yáng-Dawning formulas seem to belong squarely on the eastern horizon, just below the Green-Blue Dragon formulas, which follow in the next section of the *Fǔxíngjué*. The formulas are variations on Guìzhī Tāng, a formula whose movement is up and out, reflective of the eastern direction. Of course, the east is also where the sun rises, which is Yáng's ultimate dawning. Xiǎo Yáng Dàn Tāng 小陽旦湯 (Minor Yáng-Dawning Decoction) is mentioned in the *Jīnguì yàolüe* and is almost identical to Guìzhī Tāng. The *Fǔxíngjué* describes the presentation much like the Guìzhī Tāng presentation is described in the *Shānghánlùn*: "For treating heat effusion caused by celestial movements, with spontaneous sweating and aversion to wind, noisy breathing from the nose, and dry retching." Dà Yáng Dàn Tāng 大陽旦湯 (Major Yáng-Dawning Decoction) is very similar to Zhāng Zhòngjǐng's Xiǎo Jiàn Zhōng Tāng 小建中湯 (Minor Center-Fortifying Decoction), which is itself extrapolated from Guìzhī Tāng. In the *Jīnguì yàolüe*, Xiǎo Jiàn Zhōng Tāng is in the section on deficiency taxation. In the *Fǔxíngjué*, Dà Yáng Dàn Tāng is described this way: "To treat all cases of suffering from sweating that will not stop, with gasping breathing, generalized taxation, and physical frailness, aversion to wind and coolness, hypertonicity in the abdomen, and no interest in drinking and eating, this formula is always suitable. If the pulse is vacuous and large, it is even more of a closely fitting pattern." The more warm, light, and pungent a formula is, the more its action is upward and outward. Unlike the Qīng Lóng 青龍 (Green-Blue Dragon) formulas, along with the pungent and warm herbs shēngjiāng and guìzhī Yáng Dàn formulas contain ingredients that are sweet and/or sour, and very juicy. These herbs slow down the formulas' ascent in the east, keeping close to the transition zone on the horizon rather than further toward the south like the Qīng Lóng formulas. Another way to express this is to say that the Yáng Dàn formulas harmonize Yīn and Yáng. Dà Yáng Dàn Tāng emphasizes the enrichment of Yīn and infusing that Yīn with Yáng. Xiǎo Yáng Dàn

Tāng harmonizes Yīn with Yáng by harmonizing *yíng* Provisioning and *wèi* Defense.

The dawning of Yīn, in terms of time, is dusk. The Yīn-Dawning formulas represent the western horizon, the transition area from Yáng time to Yīn time. I place it in contrast to the Yáng Dàn formulas on the eastern horizon. The Yīn Dàn formulas resemble some well-known Shàoyáng formulas. Xiǎo Yīn Dàn Tāng is almost identical to Huángqín Tāng 黃芩湯 (Scutellaria Decoction) and, according to the *Fǔxíngjué*, is "for treating generalized heat and sweating due to celestial movements, with pain in the head and eyes, pain in the abdomen, dry retching, and diarrhea." Dà Yīn Dàn Tāng is very similar to Xiǎo Cháihú Tāng 小柴胡湯 (Minor Bupleurum Decoction) and is "a formula to treat all cases of suffering from dizziness in the head and eyes, dryness in the throat, constant tendency to dry retching, inability to get down food, vexation, and fullness in the heart, propping pain in the chest and rib-sides, and alternating cold and heat."

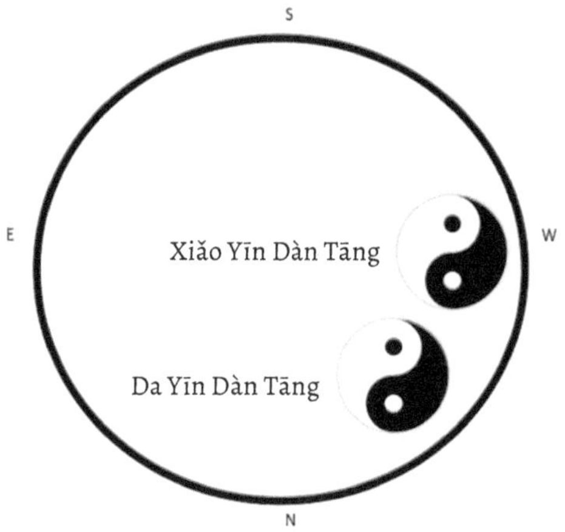

How do these formulas then relate to the western horizon? One way to think of this is to consider the direction of the ministerial fire. This is the fire that resides in the *dāntiān*, and it must burn upward. It is like a fire under a cooking pot burning upward to make soup. Yet the fire, as we have seen, comes downward into our bodies from above. To become the ministerial fire, it must pivot so that the fire can then radiate upward into the body. This pivoting action is from the Yáng conformations into the Yīn conformations. The Yángmíng is responsible for bringing the life-force Yáng down from heaven, the Shàoyáng, as a pivot, is responsible for pivoting this life-force Yáng into position and, once in place, the Shàoyīn is responsible for storing it. When I think of it this way, it makes perfect sense to situate these formulas in the west at Yīn's dawning. I have come to think of cháihú and huángqín as particular herbs for helping the Shàoyáng pivot move smoothly. Symptoms associated with these formulas are due to the heat that should be in its physiological position in the Yīn conformations stagnating as pathological heat in Yáng conformations.

5.3

The Minor and Major Formulas of the Six Spirits

The first four of these six spirits, namely the Green-Blue Dragon, White Tiger, Vermilion Bird, and Dark Warrior, represent the traditional Chinese guardian spirits of the four directions (east, west, south, and north, respectively) as well as groupings of stars in the four quadrants of the sky. The resonance of these spirits, their directions and colors, and the movements of their associated stars in the sky, with the four *zàng* organs is obvious.

The one common thread running through these formulas, besides their classical composition and the almost universal overlap with formulas from the *Shānghánlùn* that are much more widely known, is that each of them begins the list of indications with the phrase 天行 *tiānxíng*. Once again, rather than translating it here as "epidemic," as most modern translators of TCM literature would do and as may be appropriate for most contexts in medical literature from the Sòng period on, I have chosen a literal reading here as "celestial movements" because it would be ahistorical to read the later technical meaning back into this early occurrence: The Chinese characters simply mean actions, activity, or movements, in or of the sky (as a location) or Heaven (in the context of Heaven and Earth, as the complementary duality that constitutes the macrocosm, with Humanity in the middle).

I invite the reader to make up their own mind on the specific meaning of this phrase in the formulas below, but I see it here used in the sense of occurrences in the sky in the narrow sense, and in nature in general in the broader sense, since anything that happens on earth is of course due to resonance with change happening above. As such, the phrase refers to the human body failing to be in right relationship with the natural movements in the sky so that these are experienced as pathogenic as opposed to beneficial. While this could refer to weather patterns, it is also entirely appropriate to consider any other influence from the sky, most notably the movements of the stars and constellations, which the patient is not aligned with and therefore responds to by falling ill. After all, this can be the root cause of illness, just like unseasonable and pathological weather events, epidemics, or other external factors. This connection is particularly important in the following section since the titles of the formulas directly point toward the resonance between guardian spirits of the four directions, constellations of stars in the four quadrants of the sky, and the internal organs and their associated pathologies in the human body.

It is important to note again here that the phrase itself is not found in any medical texts from the classical period. In other words, it does not occur in the *Nèijīng*, *Nànjīng*, or Zhāng Zhòngjǐng's writings, or in the Mǎwángduī medical manuscripts, but only shows up with increasing frequency several centuries later. Initially used in the context of "seasonal Qì" (時氣 *shíqì*) or in a sense similar to Zhāng Zhòngjǐng's use of the phrase "cold damage" (傷寒 *shānghán*), it eventually becomes more and more strongly associated with terms like 瘟疫 *wényì*, where it really does mean "epidemic."

小青龍湯

治天行發熱惡寒，汗不出而喘，身疼痛，脈緊者方：

麻黃	三兩
杏仁（熬，打）	半升
桂枝	三兩
甘草（炙）	一兩半

上方四味，以水七升，先煮麻黃，減二升，掠去上沫，納諸藥，煮取三升，去滓。溫服八合，必令汗出徹身，不然恐邪不盡散也。

Xiǎo Qīng Lóng Tāng
(Minor Green-Blue Dragon Decoction)

A formula to treat heat effusion and aversion to cold due to celestial movements, with sweat failing to emerge and panting, generalized soreness and pain, and a tight pulse:

máhuáng	3 *liǎng*
xìngrén (slowly toasted and broken into pieces)	0.5 *shēng*
guìzhī	3 *liǎng*
gāncǎo (mix-fried)	1.5 *liǎng*

Of the four ingredients from the formula above, first decoct the máhuáng in 7 *shēng* of water until decreased by 2 *shēng*. Scoop the foam off the top, add all the other medicinals, decoct until reduced to 3 *shēng*, and remove the dregs. Take 8 *gě* per dose warm. You must cause sweat to emerge all over the body, otherwise I fear that the evil is not dispersed entirely.

Translator's Note

As anybody familiar with the *Shānghánlùn* will recognize, the present formula for Xiǎo Qīng Lóng Tāng is identical with Máhuáng Tāng from that text. The indications in that text are:

太陽病，頭痛發熱，身疼腰痛，骨節疼痛，惡風，
無汗而喘者，麻黃湯主之。

For Tàiyáng disease with headache and heat effusion, generalized soreness and lumbar pain, pain in the bones and joints, aversion to wind, absence of sweating, and panting, Máhuáng Tāng rules.

Thus, you can see how these formulas are virtually identical, even to the point of removing the foam from the decoction half-way through the cooking process, with only minor deviations in the wording.

大青龍湯

治天行，表不解，心下有水氣，乾嘔，發熱而喘咳不已者。

麻黃（去節）	
細辛	
芍藥	
甘草（炙）	
桂枝	各三兩
五味子	半升
半夏	半升
乾薑	三兩

上方八味，以水一斗，先煮麻黃，減二升，掠去上沫，內諸藥，煮取三升，去滓。溫服一升。一方無乾薑，作七味，當從。

Dà Qīng Lóng Tāng
(Major Green-Blue Dragon Decoction)

A treatment for [diseases due to] celestial movements, when the exterior fails to resolve and there is water Qì present below the heart, with dry retching, heat effusion, and panting and cough that will not stop:

máhuáng (nodes removed)	
xìxīn	
sháoyào	
gāncǎo (mix-fried)	
guìzhī	3 *liǎng* each
wǔwèizǐ	0.5 *shēng*
bànxià	0.5 *shēng*
gānjiāng	3 *liǎng*

Of the eight ingredients in the formula above, first decoct the máhuáng in 1 *dǒu* of water until decreased by 2 *shēng*. Scoop the foam off the top, add all the other medicinals, decoct until reduced to 3 *shēng*, and get rid of the dregs. Take 1 *shēng* per dose warm. An [alternate version of this] formula does not include gānjiāng and only has a total of seven ingredients. Follow that.

Translator's Note

Even more so than in the previous formula, the present formula for Dà Qīng Lóng Tāng is almost literally identical with Xiǎo Qīng Lóng

Tāng from the *Shānghánlùn*, except for the difference in name. The indications there are:

傷寒表不解，心下有水氣，乾嘔，發熱而欬，或渴，或利，或噎，或小便不利，少腹滿，或喘者，小青龍湯主之。

> *For cold damage when the exterior fails to resolve, with presence of water Qì below the heart, dry retching, heat effusion and cough, possibly thirst or diarrhea or hiccup or inhibited urination and fullness in the lower abdomen, or panting, Xiǎo Qīng Lóng Tāng rules.*

On the other hand, it is interesting that the name Dà Qīng Lóng Tāng in the *Shānghánlùn* is used for a similar formula.

Commentary by Sharon Weizenbaum

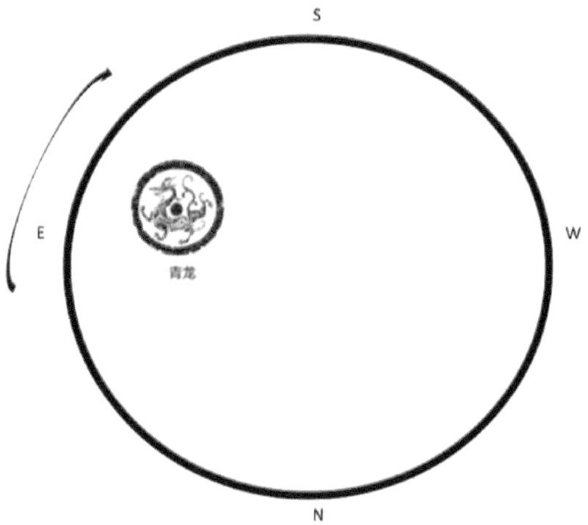

Qīng Lóng 青龍 Green-Blue Dragon –
Bringing life force Yang up and out through the east.

The Green-Blue Dragon is the spirit guardian of the east. Alignment with this quadrant generates our life-force Yáng rising toward the upper body, lungs and heart, and the body's surface. If a person's life-force is going too slow relative to the movement of the celestial bodies in this quadrant, its warmth does not fully reach completion in these locations. The Green-Blue Dragon Decoction (青龍湯 *Qīng Lóng Tāng*) formulas re-establish the right relationship with the east, which means that the formulas speed up the east to encourage the body to ascend with the eastern quadrant's timing. The *Fǔxíngjué* describes Xiǎo Qīng Lóng Tāng (Minor Green-Blue Dragon Decoction) as "A formula to treat heat effusion and aversion to cold due to celestial movements, with sweat failing to emerge and panting, generalized soreness and pain, and a tight pulse." The life-force Yáng's failure to ascend and reach the body's surface leaves the surface cold and blocked, resulting in these symptoms. The formula to speed up the body's eastern ascension is Xiǎo Qīng Lóng Tāng, which is identical to Máhuáng Tāng 麻黃湯 (Ephedra Decoction) from the *Shānghánlùn*. This formula uses the light and warm máhuáng to support the eastern function of the body's life-force.

The *Fǔxíngjué*'s Dà Qīng Lóng Tāng (Major Green-Blue Dragon Decoction) is almost identical to the *Shānghánlùn*'s Xiǎo Qīng Lóng Tāng. This formula has the same ascending and warming action as the previous formula. However, its rising action starts more deeply in the middle of the body using gānjiāng and involves pungently warming the lungs to clear cold fluids. This intensely warm and pungent method matches the body's pattern of being even slower in the east, causing it to be unable to bring warmth to the south, in this case, the upper body lungs and the surface. The *Fǔxíngjué* says that this formula is a "treatment for [diseases due to] celestial movements, when the exterior fails to resolve and there is water Qì present below the heart, with dry retching, heat effusion, and panting and cough that will not stop."

小白虎湯

治天行熱痛，大汗出不止，口舌乾燥，飲水數升不已，脈洪大者方：

石膏（綿裹）	如雞子大
知母	六兩
甘草（炙）	二兩
粳米	六合

上四味，先以水一斗，熬粳米，熟訖，去米，納諸藥，煮取六升。溫服二升，日三服。

Xiǎo Bái Hǔ Tāng
(Minor White Tiger Decoction)

A formula to treat heat and pain due to celestial movements, with great sweating that will not stop, dryness in the mouth and tongue, drinking large quantities of water without stopping, and a flooding and large pulse:

shígāo (wrapped in fine cloth)	the size of a chicken egg
zhīmǔ	6 *liǎng*
gāncǎo (mix-fried)	2 *liǎng*
jīngmǐ	6 *gě*

Of the four ingredients above, first slowly cook the rice in 1 *dǒu* of water. When it is done, remove the rice and add all the other medicinals. Decoct until reduced to 6 *shēng*. Take 2 *shēng* per dose warm, three doses a day.

Translator Note

This formula for Xiǎo Bái Hǔ Tāng is again almost literally identical with Bái Hǔ Tāng from the *Shānghánlùn*, which is there indicated for:

傷寒脈浮滑，此表有熱、裏有寒.

... a floating slippery pulse in cold damage, which means the presence of heat in the exterior and the presence of cold in the interior.

大白虎湯

治天行熱病，心中煩熱，時自汗出，舌乾，渴欲飲水，時呷嗽不已，久不解者方：

石膏（打）	如雞子大一枚
麥門冬	半升
甘草（炙）	二兩
粳米	六合
半夏	半升
生薑（切）	二兩
竹葉	三大把

上方七味，以水一斗二升，先煮粳米，米熟訖，去米，納諸藥，煮至六升，去滓。溫服二升，日三服。

Dà Bái Hǔ Tāng
(Major White Tiger Decoction)

A formula to treat heat disease due to celestial movements, with vexation and heat in the heart, periodic spontaneous sweating, a dry tongue, thirst with desire to drink water, and periodic wheezing and coughing, [all of which] have lasted a long time without resolving:

shígāo (broken into pieces)	1 piece the size of a chicken egg
màiméndōng	0.5 *shēng*
gāncǎo (mix-fried)	2 *liǎng*
jīngmǐ	6 *gě*
bànxià	0.5 *shēng*
shēngjiāng (chopped)	2 *liǎng*
zhúyè	3 large handfuls

Of the seven ingredients in the formula above, first slowly cook the jīngmǐ in 1 *dǒu* and 2 *shēng* of water. When the rice is done cooking, remove the rice, add all the other medicinals, decoct until reduced to 6 *shēng*, and remove the dregs. Take warm, 2 *shēng* per dose, three doses a day.

Translator's Note

The formula for Dà Bái Hǔ Tāng here is closely related to the formula for Zhúyè Shígāo Tāng: "For vacuity emaciation and scantiness of breath, Qì moving countercurrent, and desire to vomit, after the resolution of cold damage, Zhúyè Shígāo Tāng rules." 「傷寒解後，虛羸

少氣，氣逆欲吐者，竹葉石膏湯主之。」 The major differences are that the proportions are slightly different, that the *Shānghánlùn* calls for 3 *liǎng* of rénshēn instead of shēngjiāng, and that the *Shānghánlùn* instructs the reader to decoct the other medicinals before adding the rice, which is the reverse order from the *Fǔxíngjué*. As such we can surmise that the formulas are related but may not have shared a common source.

Commentary by Sharon Weizenbaum

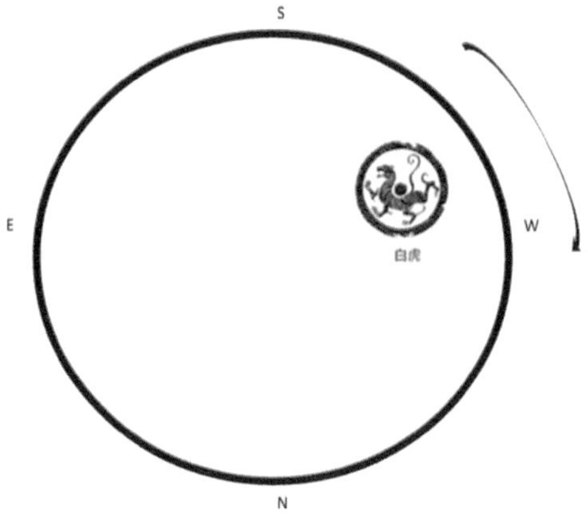

Bái Hǔ 白虎 White Tiger – Bringing life force Yang down in the west.

In the west, the guardian spirit is the White Tiger. The west's movement is downward, but unlike the southern direction that descends *toward* the west, the true west descends and dissipates toward the north. To understand the dissipation of the west, consider the characteristics of the autumn season. Autumn, corresponding to the west, comes with the decaying of fruits and the dying of leaves on the trees.

Everything in nature descends toward the ground and disintegrates. When a body fails to be in right relationship with the western direction, it fails to descend and dissipate the life-force Yáng. There is then a great deal of congested heat backing up into the south's upper body. To help the body be right with time, the *Fǔxíngjué*'s major and minor Bái Hǔ Tāng 白虎湯 (White Tiger Decoctions) use heavy, cool, pungent shígāo. Xiǎo Bái Hǔ Tāng is a "formula to treat heat and pain due to celestial movements, with great sweating that will not stop, dryness in the mouth and tongue, drinking large quantities of water without stopping, and a flooding and large pulse." It is virtually identical to the *Shānghánlùn*'s Bái Hǔ Tāng.

The *Fǔxíngjué*'s Dà Bái Hǔ Tāng is similar to its Xiǎo Bái Hǔ Tāng, without the zhīmǔ and with the addition of màiméndōng, bànxià, shēngjiāng, and zhúyè. It is closely related to the *Shānghánlùn*'s Zhúyè Shígāo Tāng. It treats the condition in which the stalling of the body in the west is even more significant, to the point that there is difficulty breathing. It is "a formula to treat heat disease due to celestial movements, with vexation and heat in the heart, periodic spontaneous sweating, a dry tongue, thirst with desire to drink water, and periodic wheezing and coughing, [all of which] have lasted a long time without resolving."

小朱鳥湯

治天行熱病，心氣不足，內生煩熱，坐臥不安，時下利純血如雞鴨肝者方：

雞子黃	二枚
阿膠	三錠
黃連	四兩
黃芩	
芍藥	各二兩

上五味，以水六升，先煮連、芩、芍三物，取三升，去滓。內膠，更上火，令烊盡，取下。待小冷，下雞子黃，攪令相得。溫服七合，日三服。

Xiǎo Zhū Niǎo Tāng
(Minor Vermilion Bird Decoction)

A formula to treat heat disease due to celestial movements, with insufficiency of heart Qì, internal generation of vexation and heat, unease whether sitting or lying down, and periodic diarrhea of pure blood like chicken or duck liver:

jīzǐhuáng	2 yolks
ējiāo	3 slabs
huánglián	4 *liǎng*
huángqín	
sháoyào	2 *liǎng* each

Of the five ingredients above, first decoct the three substances huánglián, huángqín, and shāoyào in 6 *shēng* of water until reduced to 3 *shēng*. Remove the dregs, add the ējiāo, place it back on the flame and let [the ējiāo] melt completely, then take it off the flame. Wait until it has cooled off a little and then drop in the egg yolks. Stir to combine everything. Take 7 *gě* per dose warm, three doses a day.

Translator's Note

The "vermilion bird" is also known in Chinese as 朱雀 *zhūquè*, which has basically the same meaning. The formula here is identical with Huánglián Ējiāo Tāng from the *Shānghánlùn*, in terms of the choice of medicinals, the proportions, and the instructions for preparation. The indications from the *Shānghánlùn* are:

少陰病，得之二三日以上，心中煩，不得臥，
黃連阿膠湯主之。

In Shàoyīn disease, two or three or more days after contraction if there is vexation in the heart and inability to lie down, Huánglián Ējiāo Tāng rules.

大朱鳥湯

治天行熱病，重下惡毒痢，痢下純血，日數十行，羸瘦如柴，心中不安，腹中絞急痛如刀刺方：

雞子黃	二枚
阿膠	三錠
黃連	四兩
黃芩	
芍藥	各二兩
人參	二兩
乾薑	二兩

上藥七味，以水一斗，先煮連、芩、芍、薑等五物，得四升訖，內醇苦酒二升，再煮至四升訖，去滓。次納膠於內，更上火，令烊，取下。待小冷，納雞子黃，攪令相得，即成。每服一升，日三夜一服。

Dà Zhū Niǎo Tāng
(Major Vermilion Bird Decoction)

A formula to treat heat disease due to celestial movements, with repeated malign toxic dysentery, dysentery of pure blood with several tens of bowel movements a day, marked emaciation to the point of looking like sticks and bones, inability to find ease in the heart, and wringing tense pain in the center of the abdomen as if being stabbed with a knife:

jīzǐhuáng	2 yolks
ējiāo	3 slabs
huánglián	4 *liǎng*
huángqín	
sháoyào	2 *liǎng* each
rénshēn	2 *liǎng*
gānjiāng	2 *liǎng*

Of the seven ingredients in the medicine above, first decoct the five substances huánglián, huángqín, sháoyào, gānjiāng [, and rénshēn] in 1 *dǒu* of water until you have obtained 4 *shēng*. Add 2 *shēng* of concentrated soured rice wine, decoct it again until reduced to 4 *shēng*, and remove the dregs. Next add the ējiāo to it and place it back on the flame, causing [the ējiāo] to melt, and then take it off. Wait until it has cooled off a little and then drop in the egg yolks. Stir to combine everything, and then it is done. Take 1 *shēng* per dose, three times a day and once at night.

Translator's Note

One of the earlier manuscript versions of this text, the 1975 version by Liú Déxìng 劉德興, has a slightly different version that may shed some light on this indication: Instead of the version above, it says: 治天行惡毒痢下純血日四五升。。。 "treats malign poisoning due to celestial movements, with dysentery of pure blood, 4-5 *shēng* a day...." Unfortunately, this entire section of the text is not even found at all in Zhāng Dàchāng's 張大昌 earliest manuscript version from 1974.

Commentary by Sharon Weizenbaum

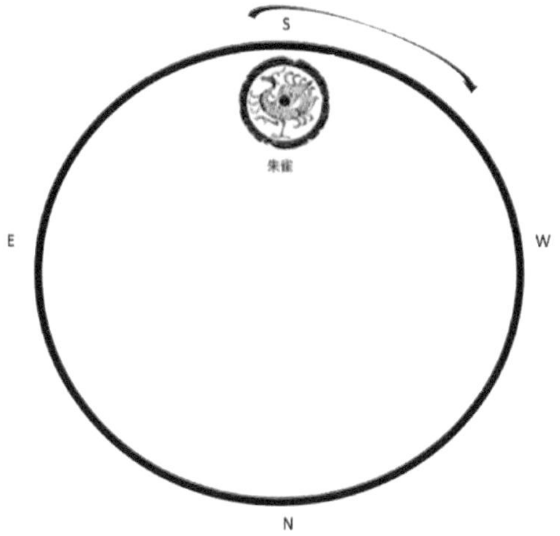

Zhū Niǎo 朱鳥 Vermillion Bird – Receiving the Shen in the Heart

Following on the Green Blue Dragon Decoction formulas in chronological order, the next two formulas are the major and minor Zhū Niǎo Tāng 朱鳥湯 (Vermillion Bird Decoction). These formulas treat conditions in which the patient's body is not in alignment with the south's guardian spirits. What does it mean for a person to be out of alignment with the south? The southern direction is the peak of heat, and it is also just beginning the turn to the west. The celestial bodies' movement traverses the southern quadrant, whose guardian spirit is Zhū Niǎo, the Vermillion Bird, but the celestial bodies never stall out. If my life-force Yáng stalls out in the south, failing to move as it should, toward the west, my body will get very hot, and my fluids will start to dry out. In this way, my body is going too slow for time. Time keeps moving from the south toward the west, but my body is stuck in the south, getting hotter and dryer. The major and minor Zhū Niǎo decoctions treat this heat by restoring the circulation of my body's life-force Yáng from the south to the west with primarily bitter cold descending herbs and juicy sweet moistening herbs. The *Fǔxíngjué*'s Xiǎo Zhū Niǎo Tāng is "a formula to treat heat disease due to celestial movements, with insufficiency of heart Qì, internal generation of vexation and heat, unease whether sitting or lying down, and periodic diarrhea of pure blood like chicken or duck liver." This formula is identical to the *Shānghánlùn*'s Huánglián Ējiāo 黄連阿膠湯 (Ephedra and Donkey Hide Glue Decoction).

Dà Zhū Niǎo Tāng is described as a "formula to treat heat disease due to celestial movements, with repeated malign toxic dysentery, dysentery of pure blood with several tens of bowel movements a day, marked emaciation to the point of looking like sticks and bones, inability to find ease in the heart, and wringing tense pain in the center of the abdomen as if being stabbed with a knife." The ingredients are the same as in Xiǎo Zhū Niǎo Tāng with the addition of rénshēn and gānjiāng, which restore the Yīn and Yáng of the middle. While the Qīng Lóng formulas use light warm, pungent herbs to restore ascension, the Zhū Niǎo formulas restore the body's relationship to the south's movement to the west with bitter cold and moistening herbs.

小玄武湯

治天行病，腎氣不足，內生虛寒，小便不利，腹中痛，四肢冷者方：

茯苓	三兩
芍藥	三兩
白朮	二兩
乾薑	三兩
附了（炮，去皮）	一枚

上五味，以水八升，煮取三升，去滓。溫服七合，日三服。

Xiǎo Xuán Wǔ Tāng
(Minor Dark Warrior Decoction)

A formula to treat disease due to celestial movements, with insufficiency of kidney Qì, internally generated vacuity cold, inhibited urination, pain in the center of the abdomen, and cold of the four limbs:

fúlíng	3 *liǎng*
sháoyào	3 *liǎng*
báizhú	2 *liǎng*
gānjiāng	3 *liǎng*
fùzǐ (blast-fried, peeled)	1 piece

Decoct the five ingredients above in 8 *shēng* of water until reduced to 3 *shēng*, and remove the dregs. Take 7 *gě* per dose warm, three doses a day.

Translator's Note

The present formula is identical with Zhēn Wǔ Tāng 真武湯 (True Warrior Decoction) from the *Shānghánlùn*. The indications are as follows: "For sweating in Tàiyáng disease, when the sweating will not resolve and this person still has heat effusion, with palpitations below the heart, dizziness in the head, convulsive twitching of the body and severe shaking to the point of almost falling to the ground, Zhēn Wǔ Tāng rules." 「太陽病發汗，汗出不解，其人仍發熱，心下悸，頭眩，身瞤動，振振欲擗地者，真武湯主之。」 It is also found in the section on Shàoyīn disease, where it is indicated as a treatment for Shàoyīn disease that has lasted for a number of days and is manifesting with "abdominal pain, inhibited urination, heaviness and pain in the four limbs, which is Water Qì..."

A note on the variation in name between Xuán 玄 ("dark") and Zhēn 真 ("true"): It is widely accepted that Xuán is the original version and that Zhēn is merely a substitution for that, based on the fact that the character 玄 was taboo for periods of the Táng and Sòng dynasties when it was part of the emperor's name and could thus not be used by anybody else. That we now think of this decoction in the context of the *Shānghánlùn* as Zhēn Wǔ Tāng is evidence that even that famous text, which we conventionally treat as solidly dating to the Hàn dynasty, has come down to us in a version that was altered centuries later. This can be seen from citations of the *Shānghánlùn* formula in other texts, such as the *Qiānjīn yìfāng* 千金翼方 (Appended Formulas Worth a Thousand in Gold), where it is listed as a formula for Shàoyīn conditions and still called Xuán Wǔ Tāng.

Lastly, it may be of interest to some readers that the wild animal associated with this spirit is the tortoise, or a mythological beast that is a combination of the tortoise and the snake.

大玄武湯

治腎氣虛疲，少腹中冷，腰背沉重，四肢清，小便不利，大便鴨溏，日十餘行，氣惙力弱者方：

茯苓	三兩
白朮	二兩
附子（炮）	一枚
芍藥	二兩
乾薑	二兩
人參	二兩
甘草（炙）	二兩

上七味，以水一斗，煮取四升。溫服一升，日三夜一服。

Dà Xuán Wǔ Tāng
(Major Dark Warrior Decoction)

A formula to treat kidney Qì vacuity and fatigue, cold in the center of the lower abdomen, heaviness in the lumbus and back, coolness in the four limbs, inhibited urination, diarrhea that looks like duck droppings with more than ten bowel movements per day, choppy Qì and weak strength:

fúlíng	3 *liǎng*
báizhú	2 *liǎng*
fùzǐ (blast-fried)	1 piece
sháoyào	2 *liǎng*
gānjiāng	2 *liǎng*
rénshēn	2 *liǎng*
gāncǎo (mix-fried)	2 *liǎng*

Decoct the seven ingredients above in 1 *dǒu* of water until reduced to 4 *shēng*. Take 1 *shēng* per dose warm, three doses a day and one at night.

Translator's Note

It is important to note that the following four formulas and the commentary ascribed to Táo Hóngjǐng at the conclusion of this section are not found in the edition of the text printed in the *Dūnhuáng zhōngyīyào quánshū*! In other words, the editors of that collection of medieval medical literature did not consider the following content authentically medieval.

The reason why they are not included there is that they are only found in some of the manuscript versions of this text, all of which date to the late 20th century to begin with. The fact that they are omitted partly or in full in many manuscript versions sheds doubts on their historicity. I have included them here for completeness' sake and for their clinical value, but encourage you to not accept them unquestioningly as part of the original *Fǔxíngjué* that was compiled as a medieval source in the centuries after Táo Hóngjǐng's death.

Commentary by Sharon Weizenbaum

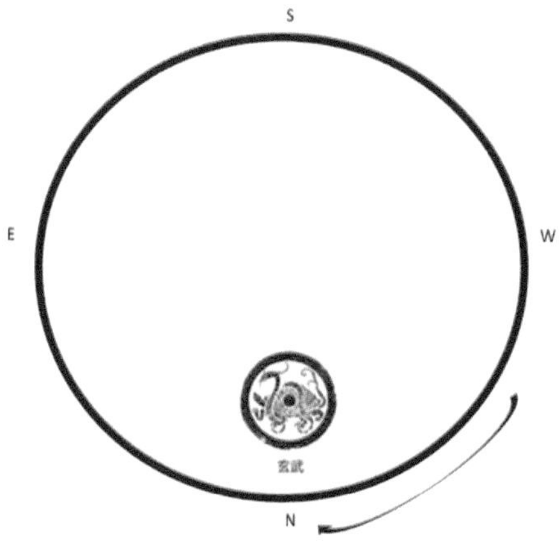

Xuán Wǔ 玄武 Dark Warrior – Submerging Yang into Yin storage

To complete the four quadrants' formulas, we go to the north's spirit guardian, the Black Turtle, who, in the image of it, is dancing with a snake. However, the formulas are not named after these animals but instead after the Dark Warrior: Xuán Wǔ 玄武. The quality of the north is one of going into the depths and storing. The turtle submerges deep into the water of the north. Our bodies must have the ability to store the life-force Yáng deeply within the north of our torso, our *dāntiān* 丹田 ("cinnabar field"). When we are not in right relationship with the north, our bodies fail to submerge and store the life-force Yáng. In this case, our bodies not only become cold due to failure to store Yáng, but cold fluids are not transformed and so accumulate easily. To restore our relationship with the north's guardian spirit, we need dense, pungent, hot herbs, like fùzǐ, as well as herbs that help us absorb and store fluids, like fúlíng and báizhú. When this lack of alignment with time is mild, Xiǎo Xuán Wǔ Tāng 小玄武湯 (Minor Dark Warrior Decoction), which is the same as Zhēn Wǔ Tāng 真武湯 (True Warrior Decoction) from the *Shānghánlùn*, is indicated. The *Fǔxíngjué* says that it is "a formula to treat disease due to celestial movements, with insufficiency of kidney Qì, internally generated vacuity cold, inhibited urination, pain in the center of the abdomen, and cold of the four limbs."

The *Fǔxíngjué* recommends *Dà Xuán Wǔ Tāng* as "a formula to treat kidney Qì vacuity and fatigue, cold in the center of the lower abdomen, heaviness in the lumbus and back, coolness in the four limbs, inhibited urination, diarrhea that looks like duck droppings with more than ten bowel movements per day, choppy Qì and weak strength." We can see that for this latter formula, the lack of alignment with the storage of the life-force Yáng is severe to the point that there is extreme leakage from below. This formula can be viewed as a combination of Zhēn Wǔ Tāng and Lǐ Zhōng Tāng 理中湯 (Center-Regulating Decoction)

小勾陳湯

治天行熱病，脾氣不足，飲食不化，腰痛下利方。

甘草	三兩
乾姜	
人參	各二兩
大棗（去核）	六枚

上四味，以水五升，煮取二升。溫分再服。

Xiǎo Gōu Chén Tāng
(Minor Hooking Array Decoction)

A formula to treat heat disease due to celestial movements, with insufficiency of spleen Qì, failure to transform food and drink, lumbar pain, and diarrhea:

gāncǎo	3 *liǎng*
gānjiāng	
rénshēn	2 *liǎng* each
dàzǎo (pitted)	6 fruits

Decoct the four ingredients above in 5 *shēng* of water until reduced to 2 *shēng*. Take warm, divided in half, in two doses.

Translator's Note

Gōu Chén "Hooking Array" is the name of a grouping of six stars that are part of the Ursa Major (Great Bear) constellation in the northern sky. Together with the "Soaring Serpent" (Téng Shé) among the Six Spirits, it belongs to Earth among the Five Dynamic Agents and is situated in the center. It is associated with the *qílín* 麒麟, the Chinese mythological "unicorn," among the six wild animals. According to the rhymed dictionary *Yùn Huì* 《韻會》 from 1297, Gōu Chén:

在天叫飛虡 鹿頭龍身；在地稱天馬。

...in Heaven is called the flying bell rack, with the head of a deer and the body of a dragon; on Earth is called the Heavenly Horse.

大勾陳湯

治天行熱病，脾氣虛，邪熱入裡，腹中雷鳴切痛，嘔吐下利不止方。

甘草	
人參	各三兩
半夏（洗，去滑）	一升
生姜（切）	二兩
黃芩	二兩
黃連	二兩
大棗（劈，去核）	十二枚

上七味，以水一斗，煮取六升。溫服二升，日三。

Dà Góu Chēn Tāng
(Major Hooking Array Decoction)

A formula to treat heat disease due to celestial movements, with spleen Qì vacuity, evil heat entering the interior, rumbling noise and cutting pain in the center of the abdomen, and retching and vomiting that will not stop:

gāncǎo	
rénshēn	3 *liǎng* each
bànxià (washed until no longer slippery)	1 *shēng*
shēngjiāng (chopped)	2 *liǎng*
huángqín	2 *liǎng*
huánglián	2 *liǎng*
dàzǎo (split and pitted)	12 fruits

Decoct the seven ingredients above in 1 *dǒu* of water until reduced to 6 *shēng*. Take warm, 2 *shēng* per dose, three times a day.

Commentary by Sharon Weizenbaum

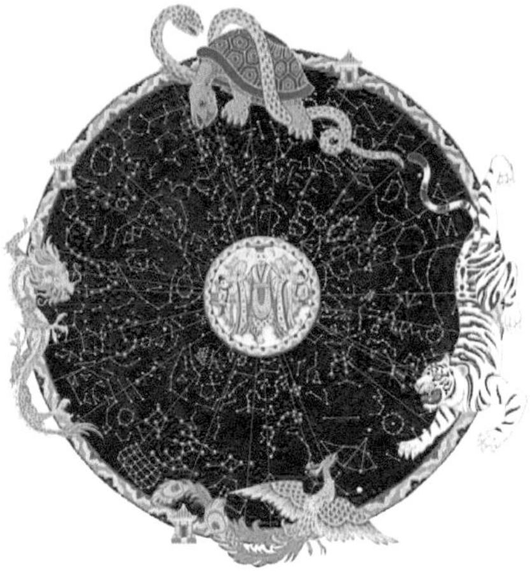

Four Directions and Pole Star

After the four directions, there is the center, which corresponds to the pole star. In heaven, the constellations move through the four quadrants around this central pole. I think it will make sense to the reader that this central area corresponds to the earth's Spleen and Stomach. They act as an axis or hub for the up and down of the circular movement of our life-force Yáng. Without the ability to pivot through this transition area, our bodies' entire cyclic motion gets jammed up. In the diagram, we see the Yellow Emperor sitting in the center, ruling over these movements. He is the yellow emperor because of his association with the central axis. The constellation that includes the group making up Gōu Chén, 勾陳, Hooking Array, is inside of the Three Enclosures (*Sān Yuán* 三垣). It rotates close to and around the north pole star. Because this position is mandrel-like, it is associated with earth, the Spleen's ascending function, and the Stomach's descending function.

The formulas, Major and Minor Gōu Chén Tāng 勾陳湯 (Hooking Array), are named after the Hooking Array asterisms that move in a circle close to and around the North Star. Xiǎo Gōu Chén Tāng uses the Middle Jiāo pungent warmth of gānjiāng to open the center and sweet moistening gāncǎo, rénshēn, and dàzǎo to nourish the soil of middle earth. The *Fǔxíngjué* considers this "a formula to treat heat disease due to celestial movements, with insufficiency of spleen Qì, failure to transform food and drink, lumbar pain, and diarrhea."

If the earth's weakness is more severe or long-lasting, there is an increase of stasis in this rotating wheel in our bodies. Our bodies then fail to match the constellations' turning around the central North Star leading to stasis in the central epigastric area. This, in turn, leads to heat. The body continues to need the pungent warmth and sweetness while also needing bitter cold yellow herbs to descend and parch stasis in the middle.

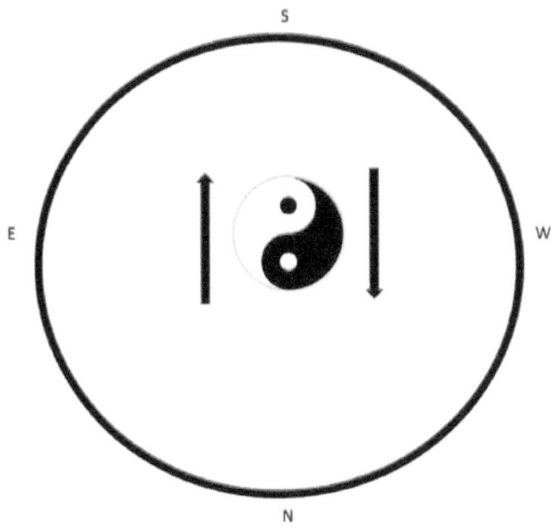

Góu Chēn 勾陳 – Hooking Array facilitating the rising and falling of the middle.

Dà Góu Chēn Tāng is very similar to the *Shānghánlùn*'s Shēngjiāng Xiè Xīn Tāng 生薑瀉心湯 (Fresh Ginger Heart-Draining Decoction). The *Fǔxíngjué* says it is "a formula to treat heat disease due to celestial movements, with spleen Qì vacuity, evil heat entering the interior, rumbling noise and cutting pain in the center of the abdomen, and retching and vomiting that will not stop." Based on the placement of this formula's action in the central area of the sky as well as in our bodies, I find it very helpful to think of these types of formulas, which are often very difficult to categorize, including Wūméi Wán 烏梅丸 (Mume Plum Pill), Bànxià Xiè Xīn Tāng 半夏瀉心湯 (Pinellia Heart-Draining Decoction), Gāncǎo Xiè Xīn Tāng 甘草瀉心湯 (Licorice Heart-Draining Decoction), Jiāo Méi Tāng 椒梅湯 (Zanthoxylum and Mume Plum Decoction) and even Zuǒ Jīn Wán 左金丸 (Left Metal Pill), as what I call Central Axis Formulas. These are all formulas that treat blockage in the middle of the body with heat and cold symptoms.

小螣蛇湯

治天行熱病，胃氣素實，邪氣不除，腹滿而喘，汗出不止方。

枳實	三兩
厚朴	二兩
甘草	二兩
芒硝	二兩

上四味，以水六升，煮取上三味至二升許，去滓，內芒硝，待熔已。頓服之。

Xiǎo Téng Shé Tāng
(Minor Soaring Serpent Decoction)

A formula to treat heat disease due to celestial movements, with constitutional repletion of stomach Qì, failure to eliminate evil Qì, abdominal fullness and panting, and sweating that will not stop:

zhǐshí	3 *liǎng*
hòupò	2 *liǎng*
gāncǎo	2 *liǎng*
mángxiāo	2 *liǎng*

Of the four ingredients above, decoct the first three in 6 *shēng* of water until reduced to about 2 *shēng*. Remove the dregs, add the mángxiāo, and wait until melted before stopping. Quaff in a single dose.

大騰蛇湯

治天行熱病，邪熱不除，大腑秘結，腹中大滿實，汗出而喘，時神昏不識人，宜此方，急下之方。

枳實	三兩
厚朴	
甘草	
大黃	
葶藶（熬黑，打如泥）	
生姜	
芒硝後下	

上七味，以水一斗二升，先煮上六味至四升，去滓，納芒硝，待熔化已。溫服二升。生姜一作大棗。

Dà Téng Shé Tāng
(Major Soaring Serpent Decoction)

To treat heat disease due to celestial movements, with failure to eliminate evil heat, constipation in the large *fǔ* organs, great fullness and repletion in the middle of the abdomen, sweating and panting, and periodic clouded spirit with failure to recognize people, this formula is suitable. Quickly drink it down.

zhǐshí	3 *liǎng*
hòupò	
gāncǎo	
dàhuáng	
tínglì (slowly toasted until black and broken up into a mud-like consistency	
shēngjiāng	
mángxiāo (added later)	2 *liǎng* each

Of the seven ingredients above, first decoct the first six in 1 *dǒu* and 2 *shēng* of water until reduced to 4 *shēng*. Remove the dregs, add the mángxiāo, and wait until it is completely melted. Take 2 *shēng* per dose warm. Instead of the shēngjiāng, an alternate [version of this] formula uses dàzǎo.

Commentary by Sharon Weizenbaum

Given that we've now covered formulas for each of the four directions plus the center, it could seem that we are complete. However, we have one more spirit formula pair to go. For me, the major and minor versions of this formula are fascinating and speak to some profound concepts in understanding the circular dynamics of Chinese medicine. In a way, the Soaring Serpent formulas, Téng Shé Tāng 騰蛇湯, pull the whole wheel of the sky together.

I hope that my commentaries so far have encouraged the reader to imagine that our body's life-force Yáng coordinates with the turning of the celestial orbs in the sky around us. Now I will go a step further to explore the mechanism at play in our bodies. It is not just that my life-force Yáng is cycling within me. My body is a mechanism for taking in influences from heaven and earth into the depths of my body, processing those influences, discarding that which is unnecessary, and turning the rest into myself as a living being. What are these "influences" that we are all receiving, processing, and expressing? From heaven, we receive Shén, which, for now, I will also call the life-force Yáng. We receive this into our hearts from the southern direction. From the south, for the life-force Yáng to enter me entirely, it must travel downwards, through the west, all the way to the north. As we've seen, the life-force Yáng submerges in the north, just as the sun is beneath us during the night. This downward movement of Yáng from heaven depends on the south's openness, the west's downward movement, and the central axis's free movement. In other words, our discussion above of the movements of the south, west, and center we can now see as important, not just for good Qì circulation, but for the very reception of life into me.

What does this have to do with the Soaring Serpent guardian spirit? What does the Soaring Serpent guard? The major and minor expressions of the Téng Shé Tāng 螣蛇湯 (Soaring Serpent

Decoctions) include herbs that purge the large intestine such as mángxiāo, zhǐshí and dàhuáng. The *Fǔxíngjué* says that Xiǎo Téng Shé Tāng is "a formula to treat heat disease due to celestial movements, with constitutional repletion of stomach Qì, failure to eliminate evil Qì, abdominal fullness and panting, and sweating that will not stop." Dà Téng Shé Tāng is a formula "to treat heat disease due to celestial movements, with failure to eliminate evil heat, constipation in the large *fǔ* organs, great fullness and repletion in the middle of the abdomen, sweating and panting, and periodic clouded spirit with failure to recognize people." Of course, these are reflections of the Chéng Qì 承氣湯 (Qì-Coordinating Decoctions) or purgative type formulas of the *Shānghánlùn*.

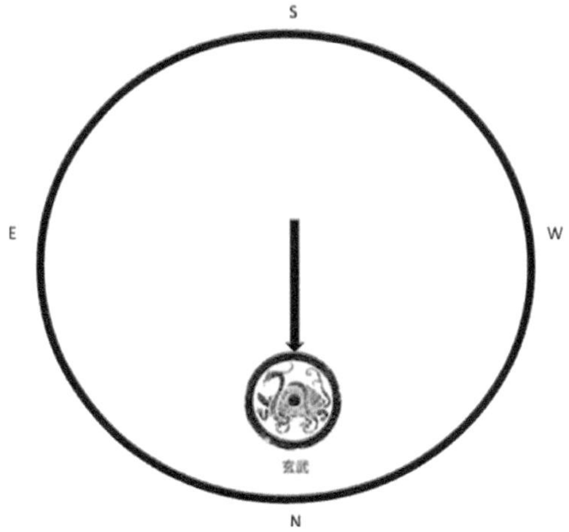

Téng Shé 螣蛇 Soaring Serpent – Bringing Yin and Yang into storage.

Here is where we revisit the fact that the northern quadrant represents two guardian spirits, the black turtle and the snake. It is essential to point out that the character translated as serpent (蛇 *shé*), is the character meaning snake. The tracts representing the pathway of the Shén (spirit) and of the life-force Yáng, from the south to the north include the Vermillion Bird of the south, the heart, the White

Tiger of the west, the lungs, and the Hooking Array, the center. The final tract along this pathway is in the large intestine, which resides in the lower torso. The large intestine is not just the body's mechanism for discharging what is not needed in the body. It is also the end stop on the pathway that allows the life-force Yáng to come down from heaven into the *dāntiān* of the body to become the *mìngmén* 命門 (Gate of Life).

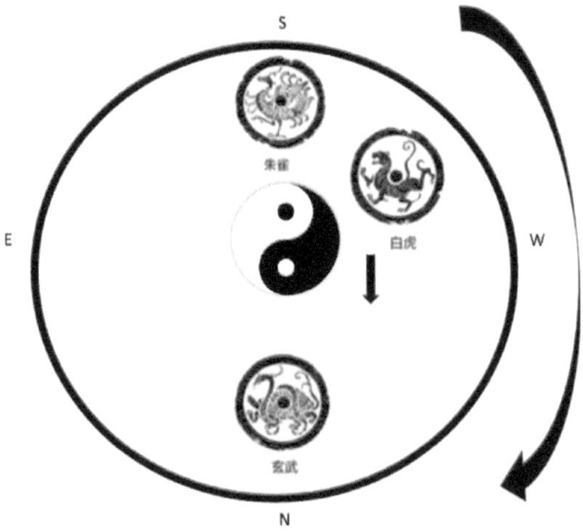

Descent of Yang

The large intestine is an organ associated with dryness. Its job is to steam moisture out of the digestate into the body. In this way, it is also a vital mechanism to receive Yīn into the body. I see this lower, northern completion of the Yángmíng, expressed by the Soaring Serpent formulas, assuring that both Yáng and Yīn enter into and achieve storage in Shàoyīn.

The Soaring Serpent group of stars is also found in the north. For me, the placement of this guardian spirit in the north illustrates the critical relationship between the lower tract of Yángmíng and the function of Shàoyīn to store Yīn and Yáng. In terms of the clinical application, a patient who needs to develop a relationship with the north's Soaring Serpent guardian spirit has a blockage in the large intestine. In this case, the treatment principle is to apply the Soaring Serpent to complete the downward movement.

弘景曰：

陽旦者，升陽之方，以黃芪為主；

陰旦者，扶陰之方，以柴胡為主；

青龍者，宣發之方，以麻黃為主；

白虎者，收重之方，以石膏為主；

朱鳥者，表滋之方，以雞子黃為主；

玄武者，溫滲之方，以附子為主。

此六方者，為六合之正精，升降陰陽，交互金木，既濟水火，乃神明之劑也。張機撰傷寒論，避道家之稱，故其方皆非正名也。但以其藥名之，以推主為識耳。

[Táo] Hóngjǐng states:

Yáng Dān (Yang Dawning) means formulas for bearing up Yáng, and they take huángqí as the ruler.

Yīn Dān (Yīn Dawning) means formulas for supporting Yīn, and they take cháihú as the ruler.

Qīng Lóng (Green-Blue Dragon) means formulas for diffusing and effusing, and they take máhuáng as the ruler.

Bái Hǔ (White Tiger) means formulas for gathering in and weighing down, and they take shígāo as the ruler.

Zhū Niǎo (Vermilion Bird) means formulas for exterior succulence, and they take jīzǐhuáng as the ruler.

Xuán Wǔ (Dark Warrior) means formulas for warming and percolating, and they take fùzǐ as the ruler.

These six formulas constitute the precise essence of the six matchings, by upbearing and downbearing Yīn and Yáng, promoting the interaction of Metal and Wood, and facilitating the mutual rescuing of water and fire. They are indeed compounds of spiritual illumination. When Zhāng Jī compiled the *Treatise on Cold Damage*, he avoided the designations of the Daoists. As such, all of his formulas are titled incorrectly. Nevertheless, he used their medicinals to name them, extrapolating their ruler to thereby recognize them.

Translator's Note

As mentioned above, this commentary is not part of the critical edition of the *Fǔxíngjué* printed in the *Dūnhuáng zhōngyīyào quánshū*. It should be noted that while Liú Déxìng's edition does not contain the two major and minor versions of these last formulas, it does include this concluding commentary by Táo Hóngjǐng. An argument against the inclusion of these formulas is that without them, and considering the two "major" and "minor" formulas as variations of a single formula in each case, the math adds up to match Táo's comment here that there are six formulas in this section, namely the two Yīn and Yáng Dawning formulas and the four guardian spirit formulas.

Commentary by Sharon Weizenbaum

We can see these formulas are named after the animals of the four directions, dawn, and dusk. Interpreting my patients' suffering in the context of their body's relationship with space/time motions has helped me understand the symptoms that arise and apply the appropriate method. I had already been seeing the structure of the *Shānghánlùn* as an expression of celestial movements when I first came across these formulas in the *Fǔxíngjué*. However, this text gives alternate names to already familiar formulas that connect them with space and time coordinates. Given that the quadrants have been named after these animals for many thousands of years, it seems likely that these formulas are very ancient and do indeed pre-date the *Shānghán zábìnglùn*.

Though I don't have concrete evidence, these names feel like the formula's true and ancient names. Given the *Huángdì nèijīng's* emphasis on the relationship of the human body's dynamics with celestial body's dynamics, I don't think it is a stretch at all to see these names as perhaps the true names. They invite an interpretation of the body as an instrument for receiving and working with heaven's influences and of the formulas as helpers in keeping this instrument in good working order. I hope the readers might look into the starry skies, at luminous dawn or a beautiful sunset, and be inspired to reflect on these great turnings.

Section Six

Emergency Treatments for Opening the Orifices

陶隱居云：

中惡卒死者，皆臟氣被壅，致令內外隔絕所致也。神仙有開五竅以救卒死中惡之方五者，錄如左：

The hermit Táo [Hóngjǐng] states:

Sudden death from being struck by malignity is in all cases due to blockage of the Qì of the *zàng* organs, which causes the inside and outside to separate. The spirit immortals have five formulas for opening the five orifices, in order to rescue people from sudden death due to being struck by malignity. They are recorded like this below:

點眼以通肝氣

治跌仆，腎腰，挫閃，氣血着滯，作痛一處，不可欠呻動轉方：

礬石燒赤，取涼冷，研為細粉，每用少許，以酢蘸，點目大眥，痛在左則點右眥，痛在右則點左眥，當大癢，螫淚大出則愈。

Eye Drops to Restore the Through-Flow of Liver Qì

A formula to treat stumbling and falling over, sudden pain from injury in the lumbar area, crippling sprains, and clinging stagnation of Qì and blood, causing pain in a single location, and inability to exhale with the mouth wide open or to turn sides:

Roast fánshí until red, let it cool off, and grind into a fine powder. Take just a small amount for each use, use vinegar to moisten it and drip it into the inner canthus of the eye. When the pain is on the left, drip it into the right canthus; when the pain is on the right, drip it into the left canthus. There will be great itching. When there is a great flow of tears as if from a poisonous insect bite, this means recovery.

吹鼻以通肺氣

治諸凡卒死，息閉不通者，皆可用此法活之。

皂角刮去皮絃，用淨肉，火上炙燥，如杏核大一塊，細辛根等分，共為極細末，每用葦管吹鼻中少許，得嚏則活也。

Nasal Insufflation to Restore the Through-Flow of Lung Qì

To treat all the various kinds of sudden death where breathing is obstructed and fails to flow through, you can use this method to bring the [patient] back to life:

Take zàojiá and scrape off the peel and strings and use only the clean flesh. Roast it over a flame until dry and take a piece the size of an apricot pit and an equal amount of xìxīn root. Process them together into extremely fine powder. For each application, take a reed tube and blow just a small amount into the nose. When you can make the patient sneeze, they will revive.

着舌而通心氣

治中惡，急心痛，手足逆冷者，頃刻可殺人。看其人唇舌青紫者及指甲青冷者是：

硝石	五錢匕
雄黃	一錢匕

上二味，共為極細末。啟病者舌着散一匕於舌下，少時即定，若有涎出，令病者隨涎咽下，必愈。

Application to the Tongue To Restore the Through-Flow of Heart Qì

To treat being struck by malignity with critical heart pain and countercurrent cold in the hands and feet, which can instantly kill the person. See whether the person has blue or purple lips and tongue and whether the nails of the fingers and toes are blue and cold, which is [the indication for the use of] this [formula]:

xiāoshí	5 *qián*-spoonfuls
xiónghuáng	1 *qián*-spoonful

Process the two ingredients above together into an extremely fine powder. Unfurl the patient's tongue and make 1 spoonful of the powder stick to the underside of their tongue. After some time, this will settle [the condition]. If there is saliva coming out and this causes the patient to swallow [the powder] down along with the saliva, this must lead to recovery.

啟喉以通脾氣

治過食難化之物，或異品有毒，宿積不消，毒勢攻注，心腹痛如刀攪。

赤小豆	
瓜蒂	各等分

共為散，每用鹹豉半升，以水二升，煮豉取一升，去滓，納散一匕，頓服。少頃當大吐則瘥。

（啟喉方：救誤食諸毒及生冷硬物，宿積不消，心中痛疼方。赤小豆、瓜蒂各等分，為散訖，加鹽豉少許，共搗為丸，以竹箸啟病者齒，溫水送入口中，得大吐即愈）。

Throat Opener to Restore the Through-Flow of Spleen Qì

To treat overeating of substances that are difficult to transform or of strange substances that contain poison, abiding accumulations that fail to disperse, the force of the poison attacking and pouring in, with pain in the heart and abdomen like a knife being twisted.

chìxiǎodòu	
guādì	equal amounts of each

Process [the two ingredients] together into a powder. For each use, take 0.5 *shēng* of salty dàndòuchǐ and decoct in 2 *shēng* of water until reduced to 1 *shēng*. Remove the dregs, add 1 spoonful of the powder, and quaff in a single dose. In a little while, there should be great vomiting. This results in recovery.

(Note: Formula for opening up the throat: A formula to rescue from erroneously having eaten the various poisons and raw, cold, and hard substances, abiding accumulations that fail to disperse, and pain in the center of the heart. Process equal amounts of chìxiǎodòu and guādì into a powder and when done, add a small amount of salty dàndòuchǐ. Pound everything together and make pills. Use a bamboo tube to open the patient's teeth, and deliver [the pill] into the patient's mouth with warm water. When you achieve great vomiting, this means recovery.)

熨耳以通腎氣

治夢魘不寐。

燒熱湯二升，入戎鹽七合，令烊化已，切蔥白十五莖納湯內。視湯再沸，即將蔥取出，搗如泥，以麻布包之，熨病者二耳，令蔥氣入耳，病者即寐也。

（灌耳方：救飲水過，小便閉塞，涓滴不通方。燒湯一斗，入戎鹽一升，蔥白十五莖，莫令蔥太熱，勺湯，指試不太熱，即灌耳中，令病者側臥，下以一盆着湯，事耳下，薰之，少時小便通，立愈。）

Ear Compress to Restore the Through-Flow of Kidney Qì

To treat nightmares and insomnia.

Boil 2 *shēng* of hot water and add 7 *gě* of róngyán. Let it dissolve completely. Then chop 15 stalks of cōngbái and add this to the decoction. See that the decoction comes back to a boil twice, and then take out the scallion. Pound it into a mud-like consistency and wrap it into a hemp cloth. Apply it with pressure as a hot compress on the patient's both ears and make the Qì of the scallion enter the ears. This will make the patient sleep.

(Formula for pouring into the ears: A formula to rescue [a patient] who has drunk too much water but whose urination is blocked with not even tiny drops coming through: Heat 1 *dǒu* of hot water and add 1 *shēng* of róngyán and 15 stalks of cōngbái. Do not let the scallions get too hot, ladle out the decoction and test with a finger to make sure it is not too hot. Now pour it into the ear. Have the patient lie on their side. Underneath place the decoction in a basin and insert this under the ear. Fumigate it, and in a little while urine will flow through. This establishes recovery.)

Reference Tables

Formulas by Pīnyīn

Pīnyīn	Chinese	English
Dà Bái Hǔ Tāng	大白虎湯	Major White Tiger Decoction
Dà Bǔ Fèi Tāng	大補肺湯	Major Lung-Supplementing Decoction
Dà Bǔ Gān Tāng	大補肝湯	Major Liver-Supplementing Decoction
Dà Bǔ Pí Tāng	大補脾湯	Major Spleen-Supplementing Decoction
Dà Bǔ Shèn Tāng	大補腎湯	Major Kidney-Supplementing Decoction
Dà Bǔ Xīn Tāng	大補心湯	Major Heart-Supplementing Decoction
Dà Bǔ Xīn Tāng	大補心湯	Major Heart-Supplementing Decoction
Dà Góu Chēn Tāng	大勾陳湯	Major Hooking Array Decoction
Dà Qīng Lóng Tāng	大青龍湯	Major Green-Blue Dragon Decoction
Dà Téng Shé Tāng	大螣蛇湯	Major Soaring Serpent Decoction
Dà Xiè Fèi Tāng	大瀉肺湯	Major Lung-Draining Decoction
Dà Xiè Gān Tāng	大瀉肝湯	Major Liver-Draining Decoction
Dà Xiè Pí Tāng	大瀉脾湯	Major Spleen-Draining Decoction
Dà Xiè Shèn Tāng	大瀉腎湯	Major Kidney-Draining Decoction
Dà Xiè Xīn Tāng	大瀉心湯	Major Heart-Draining Decoction
Dà Xiè Xīn Tāng	大瀉心湯	Major Heart-Draining Decoction
Dà Xuán Wǔ Tāng	大玄武湯	Major Dark Warrior Decoction
Dà Yáng Dàn Tāng	大陽旦湯	Major Yáng-Dawning Decoction
Dà Yīn Dàn Tāng	大陰旦湯	Major Yīn-Dawning Decoction
Dà Zhū Niǎo Tāng	大朱鳥湯	Major Vermilion Bird Decoction
Gù Yuán Bǔ Shèn Tāng	固元補腎湯	Origin-Securing Kidney-Supplementing Decoction
Jiàn Zhōng Bǔ Pí Tāng	建中補脾湯	Center-Building and Spleen-Supplementing Decoction

Pīnyīn	Chinese	English
Níng Qì Bǔ Fèi Tāng	寧氣補肺湯	Qì-Calming Lung-Supplementing Decoction
Tiáo Shén Bǔ Xīn Tāng	調神補心湯	Spirit-Attuning Heart-Supplementing Decoction
Xiǎo Bái Hǔ Tāng	小白虎湯	Minor White Tiger Decoction
Xiǎo Bǔ Fèi Tāng	小補肺湯	Minor Lung-Supplementing Decoction
Xiǎo Bǔ Gān Tāng	小補肝湯	Minor Liver-Supplementing Decoction
Xiǎo Bǔ Pí Tāng	小補脾湯	Minor Spleen-Supplementing Decoction
Xiǎo Bǔ Shèn Tāng	小補腎湯	Minor Kidney-Supplementing Decoction
Xiǎo Bǔ Xīn Tāng	小補心湯	Minor Heart-Supplementing Decoction
Xiǎo Bǔ Xīn Tāng	小補心湯	Minor Heart-Supplementing Decoction
Xiǎo Gōu Chén Tāng	小勾陳湯	Minor Hooking Array Decoction
Xiǎo Qīng Lóng Tāng	小青龍湯	Minor Green-Blue Dragon Decoction
Xiǎo Téng Shé Tāng	小螣蛇湯	Minor Soaring Serpent Decoction
Xiǎo Xiè Fèi Tāng	小瀉肺湯	Minor Lung-Draining Decoction
Xiǎo Xiè Gān Tāng	小瀉肝湯	Minor Liver-Draining Decoction
Xiǎo Xiè Pí Tāng	小瀉脾湯	Minor Spleen-Draining Decoction
Xiǎo Xiè Shèn Tāng	小瀉腎湯	Minor Kidney-Draining Decoction
Xiǎo Xiè Xīn Tāng	小瀉心湯	Minor Heart-Draining Decoction
Xiǎo Xiè Xīn Tāng	小瀉心湯	Minor Heart-Draining Decoction
Xiǎo Xuán Wǔ Tāng	小玄武湯	Minor Dark Warrior Decoction
Xiǎo Yáng Dàn Tāng	小陽旦湯	Minor Yáng-Dawning Decoction
Xiǎo Yīn Dàn Tāng	小陰旦湯	Minor Yīn-Dawning Decoction
Xiǎo Zhū Niǎo Tāng	小朱鳥湯	Minor Vermilion Bird Decoction

Pīnyīn	Chinese	English
Xiè Fèi Tāng	瀉肺湯	Lung Drain Decoction
Xiè Gān Tāng	瀉肝湯	Liver Drain Decoction
Xiè Pí Tāng	瀉脾湯	Spleen Drain Decoction
Xiè Shèn Tāng	瀉腎湯	Kidney Drain Decoction
Xiè Xīn Tāng	瀉心湯	Heart Drain Decoction
Yǎng Shēng Bǔ Gān Tāng	養生補肝湯	Life-Nurturing Liver-Supplementing Decoction
	點眼以通肝氣	Eye Drops to Restore the Through-Flow of Liver Qì
	吹鼻以通肺氣	Nasal Insufflation to Restore the Through-Flow of Lung Qì
	着舌而通心氣	Application to the Tongue To Restore the Through-Flow of Heart Qì
	啟喉以通脾氣	Throat Opener to Restore the Through-Flow of Spleen Qì
	熨耳以通腎氣	Ear Compress to Restore the Through-Flow of Kidney Qì

Formulas by English

English	Pīnyīn	Chinese
Major White Tiger Decoction	Dà Bái Hǔ Tāng	大白虎湯
Major Lung-Supplementing Decoction	Dà Bǔ Fèi Tāng	大補肺湯
Major Liver-Supplementing Decoction	Dà Bǔ Gān Tāng	大補肝湯
Major Spleen-Supplementing Decoction	Dà Bǔ Pí Tāng	大補脾湯
Major Kidney-Supplementing Decoction	Dà Bǔ Shèn Tāng	大補腎湯
Major Heart-Supplementing Decoction	Dà Bǔ Xīn Tāng	大補心湯
Major Heart-Supplementing Decoction	Dà Bǔ Xīn Tāng	大補心湯
Major Hooking Array Decoction	Dà Góu Chēn Tāng	大勾陳湯
Major Green-Blue Dragon Decoction	Dà Qīng Lóng Tāng	大青龍湯
Major Soaring Serpent Decoction	Dà Téng Shé Tāng	大螣蛇湯
Major Lung-Draining Decoction	Dà Xiè Fèi Tāng	大瀉肺湯
Major Liver-Draining Decoction	Dà Xiè Gān Tāng	大瀉肝湯
Major Spleen-Draining Decoction	Dà Xiè Pí Tāng	大瀉脾湯
Major Kidney-Draining Decoction	Dà Xiè Shèn Tāng	大瀉腎湯
Major Heart-Draining Decoction	Dà Xiè Xīn Tāng	大瀉心湯
Major Heart-Draining Decoction	Dà Xiè Xīn Tāng	大瀉心湯
Major Dark Warrior Decoction	Dà Xuán Wǔ Tāng	大玄武湯
Major Yáng-Dawning Decoction	Dà Yáng Dàn Tāng	大陽旦湯
Major Yīn-Dawning Decoction	Dà Yīn Dàn Tāng	大陰旦湯
Major Vermilion Bird Decoction	Dà Zhū Niǎo Tāng	大朱鳥湯
Origin-Securing Kidney-Supplementing Decoction	Gù Yuán Bǔ Shèn Tāng	固元補腎湯
Center-Building and Spleen-Supplementing Decoction	Jiàn Zhōng Bǔ Pí Tāng	建中補脾湯

English	Pīnyīn	Chinese
Qì-Calming Lung-Supplementing Decoction	Níng Qì Bǔ Fèi Tāng	寧氣補肺湯
Spirit-Attuning Heart-Supplementing Decoction	Tiáo Shén Bǔ Xīn Tāng	調神補心湯
Minor White Tiger Decoction	Xiǎo Bái Hǔ Tāng	小白虎湯
Minor Lung-Supplementing Decoction	Xiǎo Bǔ Fèi Tāng	小補肺湯
Minor Liver-Supplementing Decoction	Xiǎo Bǔ Gān Tāng	小補肝湯
Minor Spleen-Supplementing Decoction	Xiǎo Bǔ Pí Tāng	小補脾湯
Minor Kidney-Supplementing Decoction	Xiǎo Bǔ Shèn Tāng	小補腎湯
Minor Heart-Supplementing Decoction	Xiǎo Bǔ Xīn Tāng	小補心湯
Minor Heart-Supplementing Decoction	Xiǎo Bǔ Xīn Tāng	小補心湯
Minor Hooking Array Decoction	Xiǎo Gōu Chén Tāng	小勾陳湯
Minor Green-Blue Dragon Decoction	Xiǎo Qīng Lóng Tāng	小青龍湯
Minor Soaring Serpent Decoction	Xiǎo Téng Shé Tāng	小螣蛇湯
Minor Lung-Draining Decoction	Xiǎo Xiè Fèi Tāng	小瀉肺湯
Minor Liver-Draining Decoction	Xiǎo Xiè Gān Tāng	小瀉肝湯
Minor Spleen-Draining Decoction	Xiǎo Xiè Pí Tāng	小瀉脾湯
Minor Kidney-Draining Decoction	Xiǎo Xiè Shèn Tāng	小瀉腎湯
Minor Heart-Draining Decoction	Xiǎo Xiè Xīn Tāng	小瀉心湯
Minor Heart-Draining Decoction	Xiǎo Xiè Xīn Tāng	小瀉心湯
Minor Dark Warrior Decoction	Xiǎo Xuán Wǔ Tāng	小玄武湯
Minor Yáng-Dawning Decoction	Xiǎo Yáng Dàn Tāng	小陽旦湯
Minor Yīn-Dawning Decoction	Xiǎo Yīn Dàn Tāng	小陰旦湯
Minor Vermilion Bird Decoction	Xiǎo Zhū Niǎo Tāng	小朱鳥湯
Lung Drain Decoction	Xiè Fèi Tāng	瀉肺湯
Liver Drain Decoction	Xiè Gān Tāng	瀉肝湯
Spleen Drain Decoction	Xiè Pí Tāng	瀉脾湯

English	Pīnyīn	Chinese
Kidney Drain Decoction	Xiè Shèn Tāng	瀉腎湯
Heart Drain Decoction	Xiè Xīn Tāng	瀉心湯
Life-Nurturing Liver-Supplementing Decoction	Yǎng Shēng Bǔ Gān Tāng	養生補肝湯
Eye Drops to Restore the Through-Flow of Liver Qì		點眼以通肝氣
Nasal Insufflation to Restore the Through-Flow of Lung Qì		吹鼻以通肺氣
Application to the Tongue To Restore the Through-Flow of Heart Qì		着舌而通心氣
Throat Opener to Restore the Through-Flow of Spleen Qì		啟喉以通脾氣
Ear Compress to Restore the Through-Flow of Kidney Qì		熨耳以通腎氣

Medicinals by Pīnyīn

Pīnyīn	Chinese	Latin*	English Common Name
báizàijiāng	白截漿	Oryza sativa	fermented rice drink
báizhú	白朮	Atractylodes macrocephala	atractylodes rhizome
bànxià	半夏	Pinellia ternata	pinellia rhizome
cháihú	柴胡	Bupleurum chinense	bupleurum root
chìxiǎodòu	赤小豆	Vigna umbellata	red rice bean
cōngyè	蔥葉	Allium fistulosum	scallion leaf
dàhuáng	大黃	Rheum palmatum	rhubarb root and rhizome
dàizhěshí	代赭石	Haematitum	hematite
dàndòuchǐ	豉/淡豆豉	Glycine max	fermented soybean
dàzǎo	大棗	Zizyphus jujuba	jujube
dìhuáng	地黃	Rehmannia glutinosa	rehmannia root
ējiāo	阿膠	Equus asinus	donkey hide glue
fúlíng	茯苓	Poria cocos	poria
fùzǐ	附子	Aconitum carmichaeli	aconite prepared lateral root
gāncǎo	甘草	Glycyrrhiza uralensis	licorice root
gānjiāng	乾薑	Zingiber officinale	dried ginger
guādì	瓜蒂	Cucumis melo	muskmelon stalk
guālóu[shí]	栝楼實	Trichosanthes kirilowii	trichosanthes fruit
guìxīn	桂心	Cinnamomum cassia	shaved cinnamon bark
guìzhī	桂枝	Cinnamomum cassia	cinnamon twig
hòupò	厚朴	Magnolia officinalis	officinal magnolia bark
huánglián	黃連	Coptis chinensis	coptis rhizome

Pīnyīn	Chinese	Latin*	English Common Name
huángqí	黃芪/黃耆	Astragalus membranaceus	astragalus/vetch root
huángqín	黃芩	Scutellaria baicalensis	scutellaria/ skullcap root
jièzǐ	芥子	Brassica juncea	mustard seed
jīngmǐ	粳米	Oryza sativa	non-glutinous rice
jiǔyè	韭葉	Allium tuberosum	garlic chive
jīzǐhuáng	雞子黃	Gallus gallus	chicken egg yolk
kǔjiǔ	苦酒	Oryza sativa	soured rice wine
kǔshēn	苦參	Sophora flavescens	flavescent sophora root
lìzǐ	栗子	Castanea mollissima	chestnut
lóngdǎncǎo	龍膽草	Gentiana scabra	gentian root and rhizome
máhuáng	麻黃	Ephedra sinica	ephedra
màiméndōng	麥門冬	Ophiopogon japonicus	ophiopogon/Japanese hyacinth tuber
mángxiāo	芒硝	potassium nitrate	niter/saltpeter
mǔdānpí	牡丹皮	Paeonia suffruticosa	Tree peony/moutan root bark
rénshēn	人參	Panax ginseng	ginseng root
róngyán	戎鹽	halitum	rock salt
sháoyào	芍藥	Paeonia lactiflora/ albiflora	peony root
shēngdìhuáng	生地黃	Rehmannia glutinosa	fresh rehmannia root
shēngjiāng	生薑	Zingiber officinale	fresh ginger
shēngmá	升麻	Cimicifuga foetida/ dahurica/heracleifolia	bugbane
shígāo	石膏	Gypsum Fibrosum	gypsum

Pīnyīn	Chinese	Latin*	English Common Name
shǔjiāo	蜀椒	Zanthoxylum bungeanum	Zanthoxylum bungeanum
tínglì[zǐ]	葶藶	Lepidium apetalum or Descurainia sophia	Lepidium apetalum or Descurainia sophia
wángguāgēn	王瓜根	Trichosanthes cucumerina	snake gourd root
wǔwèizǐ	五味子	Schisandra chinensis	schisandra fruit
xiāoshí	硝石	potassium nitrate	niter/saltpeter
xièbái	薤白	Allium chinense	shallot white
xìngrén	杏仁	Prunus armeniaca	apricot seed
xiónghuáng	雄黃	realgar	realgar
xìxīn	細辛	Asarum heteropoides	asarum plant
xuánfùhuā	旋復花	Inula brittanica or lunariaefolia	Inula flower
yítáng	飴糖/黄飴	maltosum	malt sugar
zéxiè	澤瀉	Alisma plantago-aquatica	alisma rhizome
zhīmǔ	知母	Anemarrhena asphodeloides	anemarrhena root
zhǐshí	枳實	Poncirus trifoliata or Citrus aurantium	bitter orange fruit
zhīzǐ	梔子	Gardenia jasminoides	gardenia fruit
zhúyè	竹葉	Phyllostachys nigra	bamboo leaves

Medicinals by Common Name

English Common name	Pīnyīn	Chinese	Latin*
aconite prepared lateral root	fùzǐ	附子	Aconitum carmichaeli
alisma rhizome	zéxiè	澤瀉	Alisma plantago-aquatica
anemarrhena root	zhīmǔ	知母	Anemarrhena asphodeloides
apricot seed	xìngrén	杏仁	Prunus armeniaca
asarum plant	xìxīn	細辛	Asarum heteropoides
astragalus/vetch root	huángqí	黃芪/黃耆	Astragalus membranaceus
atractylodes rhizome	báizhú	白朮	Atractylodes macrocephala
bamboo leaves	zhúyè	竹葉	Phyllostachys nigra
bitter orange fruit	zhǐshí	枳實	Poncirus trifoliata or Citrus aurantium
bugbane	shēngmá	升麻	Cimicifuga foetida/ dahurica/heracleifolia
bupleurum root	cháihú	柴胡	Bupleurum chinense
chestnut	lìzǐ	栗子	Castanea mollissima
chicken egg yolk	jīzǐhuáng	雞子黃	Gallus gallus
cinnamon twig	guìzhī	桂枝	Cinnamomum cassia
coptis rhizome	huánglián	黃連	Coptis chinensis
donkey hide glue	ējiāo	阿膠	Equus asinus
dried ginger	gānjiāng	乾薑	Zingiber officinale
ephedra	máhuáng	麻黃	Ephedra sinica
fermented rice drink	báizàijiāng	白截漿	Oryza sativa
fermented soybean	dàndòuchǐ	豉/淡豆豉	Glycine max
flavescent sophora root	kǔshēn	苦參	Sophora flavescens
fresh ginger	shēngjiāng	生薑	Zingiber officinale

English Common name	Pīnyīn	Chinese	Latin*
fresh rehmannia root	shēngdìhuáng	生地黃	Rehmannia glutinosa
gardenia fruit	zhīzǐ	梔子	Gardenia jasminoides
garlic chive	jiǔyè	韭葉	Allium tuberosum
gentian root and rhizome	lóngdǎncǎo	龍膽草	Gentiana scabra
ginseng root	rénshēn	人參	Panax ginseng
gypsum	shígāo	石膏	Gypsum Fibrosum
hematite	dàizhěshí	代赭石	Haematitum
Inula flower	xuánfùhuā	旋復花	Inula brittanica or lunariaefolia
jujube	dàzǎo	大棗	Zizyphus jujuba
Lepidium apetalum or Descurainia sophia	tínglì[zǐ]	葶藶	Lepidium apetalum or Descurainia sophia
licorice root	gāncǎo	甘草	Glycyrrhiza uralensis
malt sugar	yítáng	飴糖/黃飴	maltosum
muskmelon stalk	guādì	瓜蒂	Cucumis melo
mustard seed	jièzǐ	芥子	Brassica juncea
niter/saltpeter	mángxiāo	芒硝	potassium nitrate
niter/saltpeter	xiāoshí	硝石	potassium nitrate
non-glutinous rice	jīngmǐ	粳米	Oryza sativa
officinal magnolia bark	hòupò	厚朴	Magnolia officinalis
ophiopogon/Japanese hyacinth tuber	màiméndōng	麥門冬	Ophiopogon japonicus
peony root	sháoyào	芍藥	Paeonia lactiflora/ albiflora
pinellia rhizome	bànxià	半夏	Pinellia ternata
poria	fúlíng	茯苓	Poria cocos
realgar	xiónghuáng	雄黃	realgar
red rice bean	chìxiǎodòu	赤小豆	Vigna umbellata
rehmannia root	dìhuáng	地黃	Rehmannia glutinosa
rhubarb root and rhizome	dàhuáng	大黃	Rheum palmatum

ENGLISH COMMON NAME	PĪNYĪN	CHINESE	LATIN*
rock salt	róngyán	戎鹽	halitum
scallion leaf	cōngyè	蔥葉	Allium fistulosum
schisandra fruit	wǔwèizǐ	五味子	Schisandra chinensis
scutellaria/skullcap root	huángqín	黄芩	Scutellaria baicalensis
shallot white	xièbái	薤白	Allium chinense
shaved cinnamon bark	guìxīn	桂心	Cinnamomum cassia
snake gourd root	wángguāgēn	王瓜根	Trichosanthes cucumerina
soured rice wine	kǔjiǔ	苦酒	Oryza sativa
Tree peony/moutan root bark	mǔdānpí	牡丹皮	Paeonia suffruticosa
trichosanthes fruit	guālóu[shí]	栝楼實	Trichosanthes kirilowii
Zanthoxylum bungeanum	shǔjiāo	蜀椒	Zanthoxylum bungeanum

*Note that the Latin identification in the tables refers not to the specific medicinal but only to the original plant, animal, or mineral that the medicinal is derived from. As such, guìzhī and guìxīn, for example, share the same Latin origin, Cinnamomum cassia, but differ in their English common name by the part of the plant used, namely the twig versus the bark.

Weights and Measures

Weights

1 *shǔ* 黍	=	millet grain
1 *zhū* 銖	=	10 *shǔ* 黍
1 *fēn* 分	=	6 *zhū* 銖
1 *liǎng* 兩	=	24 *zhū* 銖
1 *jīn* 斤	=	16 *liǎng* 兩

Volume

1 *dāo guī* 刀圭	=	1/10th of a square-cùn spoonful 方寸匕 *fāng cùn bǐ*
1 *cuō* 撮	=	4 *dāo guī* 刀圭
1 *sháo* 勺	=	10 *cuō* 撮
1 *gě* 合	=	2 *sháo* 勺
1 *shéng* 升	=	10 *gě* 合
1 *dǒu* 斗	=	10 *shéng* 升
1 *hú* 斛		10 *dǒu* 斗

Length

1 *cùn* 寸	=	10 *fēn* 分
1 *chǐ* 尺	=	10 *cùn* 寸
1 *bù* 步	=	5 *chǐ* 尺
1 *lǐ* 里	=	1800 *chǐ* 尺

Works Cited

1. Historical References – Alphabetical, by Pīnyīn Title

Bèijí qiānjīn yàofāng 《備急千金要方》 (Essential Formulas Worth a Thousand in Gold to Prepare for Emergencies). Sūn Sīmiǎo 孫思邈, 652.

Běncǎo gāngmù 《本草綱目》 (Classified Materia Medica). Lǐ Shízhēn 李時珍, 1596.

Běncǎo yǎnyì 《本草衍義》 (Expanded Meaning of the Materia Medica). Kòu Zōngshì 寇宗奭, 1116.

Dàodéjīng 《道德經》 (Classic of the Way and its Virtue-Power). Attributed to Láozi, Zhōu period.

Huángdì nèijīng 《黃帝內經》 (Yellow Emperor's Inner Classic). Anon., Hàn period.

Ishimpō 《醫心方》 (Formulas from the Heart of Medicine). Tanba no Yasuyori, 984.

Jīnguì yàolüè 《金匱要略》 (Essentials from the Golden Cabinet). Zhāng Zhòngjǐng 張仲景, Hàn period. The second half of the *Shānghán zábìng lùn*.

Língshū 《靈樞》 (Magic Pivot). Anon., Hàn period. The second half of the *Huángdì nèijīng*.

Màijīng 《脈經》 (Pulse Classic). Wáng Shūhé 王叔和, late third century CE.

Nànjīng 《難經》 (Classic of Difficulties). Anon, Hàn period.

Nǚkē bǎiwèn 《女科百問》 (Hundred Questions on Gynecology). Qí Zhòngfǔ 齊仲, 1220 CE.

Qiānjīn yìfāng 《千金翼方》(Appended Formulas Worth a Thousand in Gold). Sūn Sīmiǎo 孫思邈, 682.

Shānghánlùn 《傷寒論》 (Treatise on Cold Damage). Zhāng Zhòngjǐng 張仲景, Hàn period. The first half of the *Shānghán zábìng lùn*.

Shānghán zábìng lùn 《傷寒雜病論》 (Treatise on Cold Damage and Miscellaneous Diseases). Zhāng Zhòngjǐng 張仲景, Hàn period.

Shénnóng běncǎo jīng 《神農本草經》 (Divine Farmer's Classic of Materia Medica). Anon., Hàn period.

Shénnóng běncǎojīng jízhù 《神農本草經輯注》 (Collected Commentaries on the Divine Farmer's Classic of Materia Medica). Táo Hóngjǐng 陶弘景, ca. 500 CE.

Shuōwén jiězì 《說文解字》 (Explaining Characters and Analyzing Characters). Xǔ Shèn 許慎, 2nd century CE.

Sùwèn 《素問》 (Plain Questions). Anon., Hàn period. The first half of the *Huángdì nèijīng*.

Wàitái mìyào 《外台秘要》 (Essential Secrets from the Outer Terrace/Palace Library). Wáng Tāo 王燾, 752.

Yìjīng 《易經》 (Classic of Changes). Anon., Zhōu period.

Yīshuō 《醫說》 (Explanations of Medicine). Zhāng Gāo 張杲, 1189.

Yìwénzhì 《藝文志》 (Treatise on Literature), early second century CE.

Zhēnjiǔ jiǎyǐjīng 《針灸甲乙經》 (A-Z Classic of Acupuncture and Moxibustion). Huángfǔ Mì Mì 皇甫謐, ca. 260 CE.

Zhōngcángjīng 《中藏經》 (Classic Stored in the Center). Anonymous, medieval period.

Zhōu Yì Xìcí 《周易繫辭》(Appendix on the Yìjīng). Anonymous, Warring States.

Zhǒuhòu bèijífāng 《肘後備急方》 (Formulas to Prepare for Emergency to Keep up one's Sleeve). Gě Hóng 葛洪, early fourth century CE.

Zhūbìng yuánhòu lùn 《諸病源候論》 (Discourse on the Origins and Signs of the Various Diseases). Cháo Yuánfāng 巢元方, 610 CE.

2. Contemporary References – Alphabetical by Author

Bensky, Dan, Steven Clavey, Erich Stoger, and Andrew Gamble, *Chinese Herbal Medicine: Materia Medica*. Eastland Press, 1990 and 2004.

Cóng, Chūnyǔ 從春雨, ed., *Dūnhuáng zhōngyīyào quánshū* 《敦煌中醫藥全書》 (Complete Collection of Chinese Medical Manuscripts from Dūnhuáng). 中醫古籍出版社, 1994.

Despeux, Catherine, "The System of the Five Circulatory Phases and the Six Seasonal Influences" in Elisabeth Hsu, ed., *Innovation in Chinese Medicine*. Cambridge University Press, 2001, pp. 121-165.

Féng Shìlún 馮世綸, *Zhōngguó tāngyè jīngfāng: Shānghán zábìnglùn chuánzhēn* 《中國湯液經方：傷寒雜病論傳真》 (Classical Formulas for Decoctions from China: The True Transmission of the *Treatise on Cold Damage and Miscellaneous Diseases*). 人民軍醫出版社, 2005.

Gläser, Abel, transl., *Tao Hong-jing, Fu Xing Jue. Procédés subtils des Mouvements de l'Etoile Alcor*. Institut Liang Shen de Médecine Chinoise, 2019.

Harper, Donald, *Early Chinese Medical Literature: The Mawangdui Medical Manuscripts*. RoutledgeCourzon, 2015.

Lo, Vivienne, and Penelope Barrett, eds, *Imagining Chinese Medicine*. Brill, 2018.

Lo, Vivienne, and Christopher Cullen, eds., *Medieval Chinese Medicine: The Dunhuang Medical Manuscripts*. RoutledgeCourzon, 2005.

Mǎ, Jīxìng 馬繼興, *Dūnhuáng gǔyījí kǎoshì* 敦煌古醫籍考釋 (Philological Study of the Ancient Dūnhuáng Medical Records). 江西科學技術出版社, 1988.

Mǎ, Jīxìng et als., *Dūnhuáng yīyào wénxiàn jíjiào* 敦煌醫藥文獻輯校 (Collected Collations of the Medical Texts from Dūnhuáng). 江西科學技術出版社, 1998.

Muller, Charles, "The Emergence of Essence-Function 體用 Hermeneutics in the Sinification of Indic Buddhism," in *Fójiàoxué* 佛教學 (Buddhist Studies) 19 (June 2016).

Unschuld, Paul U., *Huang Di Nei Jing: Nature, Knowledge, Imagery in an Ancient Chinese Medical Text*. University of California Press, 2003.

Unschuld, Paul U., *Medicine in China: A History of Pharmaceutics*. University of California Press, 1986.

Wang, Jiqing, "Aurel Stein's Dealings with Wang Yuanlu and Chinese Officials in Dunhuang in 1907," in *International Dunhuang Project News* 30, pp. 1-6.

Wang, Shumin, "*Tangye jingfa*: A lost text in the *Hanshu* bibliography," in Vivienne Lo and Christopher Cullen, eds., *Medieval Chinese Medicine: The Dunhuang Medical Manuscripts*. RoutledgeCourzon, 2005, pp. 322-344.

Wáng, Xuětái 王雪苔, *Fǔxíngjué zàngfǔ yòngyào fǎyào jiàozhù kǎozhèng* 《辅行诀脏腑用药法要》 校注考证 (A textual analysis of *Fǔxíngjué zàngfǔ yòngyào fǎyào*, collated and annotated). 人民军医出版社, 2008.

Weizenbaum, Sharon, "What does 經 mean?," blog post published at https://whitepinehealingarts.org/what-does-經-mean/.

Wilms, Sabine, *The Divine Farmer's Classic of Materia Medica*. Happy Goat Productions, 2017.

Wilms, Sabine, *Channeling the Moon: A Translation and Discussion of Qí Zhòngfǔ's* Hundred Questions on Gynecology, Parts One and Two. Happy Goat Productions, 2019 and 2020.

Wiseman, Nigel, and Ye Feng, *Practical Dictionary of Chinese Medicine.* Paradigm Publications, 2014.

Yáng, Shìyǐn 楊師尹, *Yī Yǐn Tāngyèjīng 伊尹湯液經* (Yī Yǐn's Classic of Decoctions). 一錢閣, 1948.

Zhāng, Dàchāng 張大昌 and Qián Chāochén 錢超塵, *Fǔxíngjué wǔzàng yòngyào fǎyào chuánchéngjí* 《辅行诀五臟用药法要》 傳承集 (Collected Transmissions of *Fǔxíngjué wǔzàng yòngyào fǎyào*). 學苑出版社, 2008.

Zhāng, Qíchéng 張其成, "Wǔzàng liùfǔ bǔxiètú jiěshuō 五臟六腑補瀉圖解說" (Explaining the illustrations for supplementing and draining of the five *zàng* and six *fǔ* organs), in Wáng Shūmín 王淑民 and Vivienne Lo, *Xíngxiàng zhōngyī* 《形象中醫》 (Visualizing Chinese Medicine). 人民衛生, 2007, pp. 175-181.

Index

D

E

F

G

H

I

J

K

L

M

N

O

P

Q

R

S

T

U

V

W

X

Y

Z

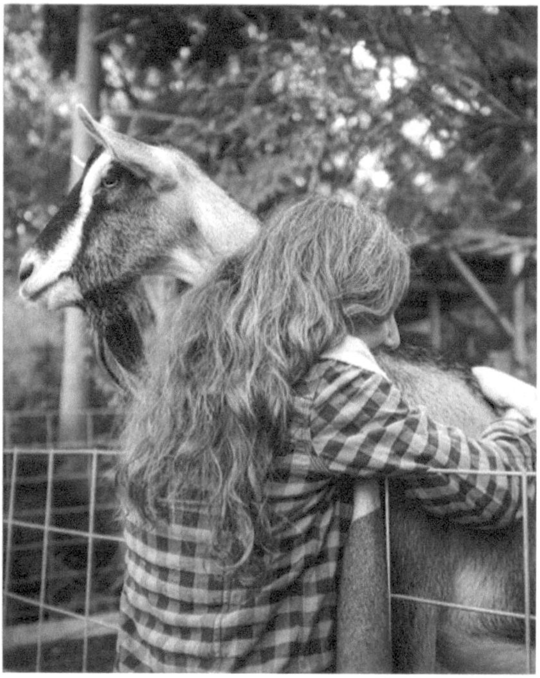

www.ingramcontent.com/pod-product-compliance
Ingram Content Group UK Ltd.
Pitfield, Milton Keynes, MK11 3LW, UK
UKHW041646011026
15471UKWH00018B/74

9 781732 157170